A U T I S M

Prevention, Care, and Management

The Plight of the Canary Children

and Their Release from Captivity

Marvin D. Anderson, M.D.

Foreword by Sandra Cabot, M.D.

Introduction by Stephanie Cave, M.D., FAAFP

G.U.D. Publishers
Cedar, MI

A U T I S M

Prevention, Care, and Management

D i s c l a i m e r

Autism, Prevention, Care, and Management is based on sources believed to be accurate and reliable, and every reasonable effort has been made to make the book as complete and accurate as possible. However, total completeness and accuracy are not guaranteed.

Although *Autism,Prevention, Care, and Management* discusses the detection of autism spectrum disorders as well as various alternative systems of medical management, it is intended only as a general introduction to these topics. It is not meant to give specific recommendations or medical, psychological, or other life advice, nor does it make any warranties or guarantees of any sort that any of the information in the book (or information in any of the books, material, or services of any practitioner recommended within this book) will produce any particular medical, physical, emotional, or other result.

There is no confidential, professional, or other relationship between the reader and the author or publisher created as a result of the information provided in *Autism, Prevention, Care, and Management* as a result of an e-mail or other forms of communication between the reader and the author or the publisher. G.U.D. Publishers or Marvin D. Anderson, M.D. will not be liable to the reader or any other party for direct or indirect compensatory, special, incidental, or consequential damages.

Library of Congress Cataloging Number: 2012947087

ISBN: 978-0-9858650-0-9
Printed in the U.S.A. by Allegra Printing, Traverse City, MI, 49686

Dedicated to the Parents

of Children with Autism

This little book is so important that it belongs on the kitchen table. It merits this place, rather than on a bookshelf, so that all parents and parents-to-be can quickly read and absorb its critical message. The author discusses the suspected causes, management, and prevention of the modern plague of autism and related conditions, such as Asperger's Syndrome, Attention Deficit Disorder (ADD), and Attention Deficit Hyperactivity Disorder (ADHD). Once parents and parents-to-be understand the crucial principles set forth in these pages, they must aggressively take action to protect and nurture their existing and future children who cannot protect themselves.

C O N T E N T S

F o r e w a r d

by

Sandra Cabot, M.D.

Dr. Cabot is world-renowned medical author. She has written more than twenty books on health-related issues. Her best-selling book, entitled The Liver Cleansing Diet, has sold over two million copies and has been translated into five languages. Her website is www.liverdoctor.com.

Dr. Marvin Anderson has written a book that will serve as a lifeline to the thousands of parents who care for children with autism. Dr. Anderson is eminently qualified to write this book, as he is a true academic who is Board Certified in Internal Medicine and in Nutrition. As well as being an academic, he has extensive clinical experience, and the ability to take the complex subject of autism and make it understandable for the average person.

The dedication and passion of Dr. Anderson and his colleague, Dr. Stephanie Cave, are truly inspiring, along with their years of hard work. Such effort can now become a gift in the form of this book to the parents of children with autism.

Prevention of autism

I believe that the prevention of autism begins well before conception. While no human being has a perfect set of chromosomes, or genes, we can improve our genetic inheritance and that of our offspring. Through good nutrition we can repair and diminish many genetic faults and imperfections we may have inherited and accumulated over our lifetimes. These genetic imperfections lie in our eggs (follicles) and sperm and are passed onto our offspring. By repairing these faults, we can prevent passing them onto our offspring and reduce the chances of autism. We can also reduce the risk of our offspring developing cancer or immune dysfunction during childhood.

How do we repair genetic faults?

- We must ensure we are not deficient in selenium, and the best way to do this is to take a supplement of selenomethionine in a dose of 100 mcg daily.

- We must avoid vitamin D deficiency by getting regular sunshine and checking our serum vitamin D levels. If they are low, take a supplement of vitamin D3.

- We must consume foods high in:

  Folic acid, especially green leafy vegetables

  Vitamin C present in citrus, bell peppers and berries

  Vitamin E (avocados are the best source)

  Iodine, such as kelp or iodized salt; take an iodine supplement

Omega 3 essential fatty acids by taking fish oil liquid (Carlson's is a good brand), ground flaxseeds, chia seeds, and walnuts

- We must also help our livers to detoxify our bodies from petrochemicals and heavy metals, as these things cause damage to our chromosomes. This can be achieved by taking a good liver formula containing the herb Milk Thistle, taurine, cysteine, glutamine, and B vitamins. The liver requires the mineral sulfur to detoxify our bodies. Foods high in sulfur, such as garlic, onions, and cruciferous vegetables (such as broccoli, cabbage, cauliflower and Brussels sprouts), should be consumed regularly.

It is an excellent idea to check your family history by tracing back three generations (your parents, grandparents, and great grandparents) to look for cases of autism and hyperactivity or delayed development. Look for severe allergies, gluten intolerance, and autoimmune diseases. If a strong family history of these ailments is present, follow the program outlined above and try to repair these potentially inheritable faults. If you have the luxury, try to seek the counsel of a doctor who specializes in genetic diseases before you try to conceive a child.

Be careful with childhood vaccinations

If there is a family history of autism, delayed development, severe allergies, or autoimmune disease, try to seek the services of a holistic doctor who understands nutritional medicine. This is because you will need to be extremely careful when you vaccinate your children.

You may need to prepare your child with nutritional supplements in liquid form before any vaccinations are given. Through breastfeeding, you can prepare your infant by taking the correct supplements yourself.

You may need to avoid giving your child a course of multiple vaccines in one hit. This has become standard practice today. Instead, it may be safer to give only the most important vaccinations, such as tetanus and polio, in staggered doses and not concurrently. Rubella can be given at the onset of puberty. Children who are gluten intolerant will often not respond to a vaccination against hepatitis B. (1, 2)

Never vaccinate your child if he/she has a fever or an infection. It is also not wise to vaccinate while your child is on antibiotic drugs or just after having taken antibiotic drugs, as these drugs reduce the ability of your child's immune system to cope with a vaccine.

Breastfeeding is best

Try to breast feed your child, as this will reduce the risk of allergies and autoimmune disease. Breast feeding also confers significant immunity against common infections while your child is on breast feeding. Make sure your diet is good with plenty of raw fruits and vegetables, and eggs. Take supplements of iodine, selenium and omega 3 essential fatty acids, as these substances will come through your breast milk to your infant. The first 12 months of life are critical for brain development and these supplements are able to optimize the growth of neurological pathways and brain mass.

The autoimmune connection

A study has found that women with an autoimmune disease are up to three times more likely to have a child with autism than the general population. The autoimmune diseases included in this study were celiac disease, Type I diabetes, and rheumatoid arthritis. (3)

Celiac disease is an autoimmune disease whereby ingestion of gluten causes damage to the lining of the small intestine. This can cause digestive problems, such as bloating and diarrhea. However, many cases of celiac disease cause no digestive symptoms at all, yet damage to the body still occurs.

Autoimmune diseases are extremely common and they are more common in women than in men.

Research carried out at the Johns Hopkins University collected data on 3,325 Danish children diagnosed with autism spectrum disorder. The children were born between 1993 and 2004. The data showed that women with autoimmune diseases are more likely to have a child diagnosed with autism. The increased risk for mothers with Type 1 diabetes was a little less than double; for rheumatoid arthritis it was 1.5 times, but for celiac disease it was three times greater.(3)

Autoimmune diseases cause a great deal of inflammation and tissue damage in the body. The inflammation can affect the development of the fetus while in its mother's uterus. Women with celiac diseases are more prone to giving birth prematurely and having small birth weight babies. Both of those factors are associated with an increased risk of autism.

Autism is thought to be an immune disorder (rather than a brain disorder), and this study further confirms this belief. Approximately 80 percent of our immune system is located in your digestive tract. Therefore, digestive problems affect the immunity as a whole and your children's immunity as well, when you become pregnant.

Luckily, a lot can be done to correct immune system dysfunction and overcome autoimmune diseases. The Danish study referred to undiagnosed or untreated celiac disease. If a celiac patient sticks to a gluten-free diet 100 percent of the time and addresses nutritional deficiencies that go hand in hand with the condition, her offspring are not at increased risk of autism due to the presence of her celiac condition.

We actually recommend that anybody with an autoimmune condition avoid all gluten and cow's milk, regardless of the specific type of autoimmune disease. These dietary changes, combined with the right nutritional supplements, are extremely successful in the treatment of autoimmune diseases.

You can get improvement

We have talked about prevention, but just as important is improving a child with autism. The brain is a "plastic organ" in the sense it can change shape and size and grow new pathways, while redirecting wrong ones. While the brain is still young, we must seize the opportunity to do this by using Dr. Anderson's methods, along with correct nutritional supplementation. The inflammation attacking the brain of a child with autism can be reduced and result in subsequent improvement in all aspects of mental and emotional behavior of the child. With persistence and patience, huge improvement can be seen after 6 to 12 months.

In summary, I would like to thank a few people:

Firstly, Dr. Anderson, who is so nice to have as a colleague and friend, and who, despite his hugely academic background, is immensely humble.

Secondly, I thank the parents of children with autism, because I truly admire you. You are amazing and I think you need a medal of honor! You have a big load to bear, probably much bigger than I will ever know, as I do not have a child with autism. I am sure you will need all the help you can get along the way, and Dr. Anderson is someone who, with the grace of God, can truly help you on your journey. His book will enable this understanding.

Sandra Cabot, M.D.

Sydney, Australia and Phoenix, AZ, USA

1) McMahon BJ, Dentinger CM, Bruden D, et al Antibody levels and protection after hepatitis B vaccine; results of a 22-year follow-up study and response to a booster dose. J Infectious Dis. 2009; 200(9):1390-1396.

2) Leonardi S, Spina M, Spicuzza L, Rotolo N, LaRosa M. Hepatitis B vaccination failure in celiac disease: is there a need to reassess current immunization strategies? Vaccine 2009;27(43):6030-6033. E Pub 2009 Aug 12.

3)Atladottir HO, Pedersen MG, Thorsen P, et al. Association of Family History of Autoimmune Diseases and Autism Spectrum Disorders. *Pediatrics.* 2009;124(2):687-694. EPub 2009 July 5.

Introduction

by

Stephanie Cave, M.D., FAAFP

Dr. Cave has cared for over 10,000 persons with autism. She is the author of the now classic book involving the care of children entitled What Your Doctor May Not Tell You About Childhood Vaccinations. *As a medical practitioner, I have learned much from Dr. Cave. Her compassion, her moral rectitude, her practicality, and her wisdom are goals we all strive for but which she has in great measure already achieved. mda*

I have spent the last sixteen years of my life treating children in the Autism spectrum. Researchers have tried to prove that this is a purely genetic problem, but it is not possible to have a genetic epidemic. The whole gene pool would have to change for this to occur. There is no denying a genetic predisposition to autism exists, and that many genes are involved, including those coding for methylation.

The environment certainly plays a significant part in triggering the autism process. Several theories have been suggested, including a relationship between the evidence of a connection with heavy metals, such as ethyl mercury and aluminum, and the onset of autistic behavior in children. Heavy metal as an environmental trigger is biologically plausible. The Institute of Medicine, however, has concluded that there is not significant evidence of a connection between heavy metal and autism.

Theresa Deisher, PhD, has suggested that spikes in the incidence of autism correspond with the introduction and continued use of human tissue in vaccines. She offers the explanation that the human DNA in the vaccine can recombine with the DNA of the child being vaccinated in areas on the gene that affect nerve synapse function and mitochondrial function The children who cannot methylate are the potential targets of such a recombination. Her theory is biologically plausible, but research money is not available for topics like this.

The altered food sources in the world are part of the problem. Food is grown in depleted soil and pesticides are used on the crops. Supplements become a necessity, if health is the goal. Animals in the food chain are grain-fed instead of being range-fed. Chickens are housed in massive buildings in crowded surroundings and arsenic is added to their food. Fish are fed grain in fish farms, making them sources of omega 6 oil, rather than omega 3 oil.

The GI tract becomes a target of entry for many invaders from the environment through the permeable wall in the tract. Undigested food, bacteria, yeast, viruses, chemicals, and metals find their way into the bloodstream of the children. They are left with chronic pain, until the GI tract is balanced with good flora.

Plasticizers are in food, water, and even in breast milk. Insecticides are sprayed in houses where children are living.

We live in a "wireless" environment and use cell phones and lap top computers around children. Do we know the real effect of these on the human brain, particularly the child's brain? To treat autism effectively, a team approach is necessary. Treatment of the GI tract is a starting point. For the diets of families, organic foods grown in a nutrient-based soil are better than store-bought foods grown with pesticides. Beneficial bacteria are strengthened in growth through the use of probiotics. Cellular chemistry should be corrected. Heavy metals should be removed from the child's biochemical make up. Mitochondrial function needs to be strengthened, if it is weak. Therapies, such as Applied Behavioral Analysis, speech therapy, and occupational therapy work in tandem with the metabolic approaches to treatment. Dr. Anderson's book has information about all of these modes of therapy, and more. His dedication to the children and their families shines through the pages of this book. Improvement and recovery for the children in the spectrum are his goals for the families and practitioners.

Stephanie F. Cave, M.D., M.S., FAAFP

Baton Rouge, Louisiana

Acknowledgments

On a summer evening many years ago, I saw a speechless little boy in the emergency room. He probably had autism. I didn't know how to help him. I probably still wouldn't know, were it not for the generous help and self-sacrifice of long-time friends, Peter Christopher Gruters, Dr. Paul Faucher, and Dr. and Mrs. Douglas Wigton.

Nearly two years ago, Peter suggested I write this book. He has helped me almost daily with its composition and editing. Paul sent one reference book after the other. Over the decade we practiced together, Dr. Wigton worked doubly hard to allow me to take the additonal time with my patients. And our main editors, Lou and nurse Mary Jo Rubino have labored tirelessly and have good-heartedly weathered many revisions.

In addition, my special gratitude goes to those who took time to read portions or all of the manuscript and to offer comments and criticism, Although the final responsibility for the accuracy and validity of the text is mine, I could not have completed this book without the skilled help of the following friends and associates:

Editors: Kelly Trumble, PhD, Capt. Terrence Gruters, USAF, Sandra Cabot, M.D., Stephanie Cave, M.D. M.S. FAAFP,

Terry J. Baumann, Pharm.D., Diane Kobus, M.S., Prof. Don Huber of Purdue University (ret'd), Larry Newman, Liz Mumper, M.D.,FAAP, Stephen Olmstead, M.D. Susan Costen Owens, M.S., Robert David, PhD, David Quigg, PhD, Patrick Hanaway, M.D., Treya Palmer, N.D., Joanne A. Balog; and Jacquelyn J. Kaschel of PEACE Ranch.

Additional support and information were provided by my wonderful wife, Jill Anderson, RN, MSN, PNP, Kris Zimmerman, D.O for electronic technical support, Nicole Lee Anderson, our daughter, for cover design, Prof. H.M. "Skip" Kingston of Duquense University, Matt Pamuku, the Munson Hospital Medical Sciences Library, the Autism Research Institute, Murray Bast, William Rutherford, Capt. Guy Gruters, USAF, Timothy Axe, Daniel and Justin Soutar, Theresa McClure, Michael Burkhardt, Aaron and Valerie Byrnes, John F. Twomey, Jr., Terrence Weber; and Roger Hughes.

Finally, I gratefully acknowledge my indebtedness to a host of wonderful people from years past who have taught me not only how to write but also how to live: The instructors in physics and classical languages at the University of Detroit Jesuit High School, Dr. Joseph Duffy of the English Department of the University of Notre Dame, Dr. Robert Coffey of the Department of Surgery of Georgetown University School of Medicine, Dr. Hans Falk of the Carcinogenesis Branch of the National Cancer Institute, Dr. Herbert S. Rosenkranz of the Department of Microbiology of the Columbia University College of Physicians and Surgeons, and Dr. Robert K. Nixon of the Department of Internal Medicine of Henry Ford Hospital in Detroit.

If this book should make an impact on the scourge of autism, credit will go to all the inspiration and guidance from which I have benefitted and not at all to any efforts of my own.

Preface

There are many excellent books written about autism. These are well-referenced, in-depth presentations of information about predisposing conditions and management strategies. However, these books are oftentimes written for individuals who are either experts or very familiar with autism and its related disorders. They are generally very thorough, quite complex, often specialized in topic, and not inexpensive. This book, on the other hand, has been primarily written for the novice and the non-professional. Its goal is to provide a clear and inexpensive overview of the causes, current management, and suggestions for the prevention of autism. Its purpose is to sound the alarm for parents and caregivers, and to motivate them to take action.

GOALS

This book has two specific missions. The first is to help parents prevent their future children from developing autism. The second mission is to help parents and other caregivers to provide the best possible treatment for any of their children or charges who already suffer from autism.

KEEP IT SIMPLE

By design, the book is short, so that it can be read and understood in an evening or over a weekend by parents and other caregivers, even if they haven't previously studied the autism topic.

FRIENDLY STYLE

The format is largely conversational and is based on my experience, research, and training. In line with this approach, I have minimized the use of quotations and references . However, for those who wish to study further, more detailed and additional information can be accessed from the sources that are cited in the References section.

WHAT IS AUTISM, ANYWAY?

We can begin by stating that autism is a disorder from normal development and is identified by its neurological effects on affected individuals. These neurological effects, as we will see later, are closely tied to gastrointestinal functions. They vary and usually include one or more of the following: the delay of or the absence of language, impaired communication, lagging socialization, and/or repetitive behavior. Such behavior, oftentimes termed "stimming", differs for each child, and varies, depending on the circumstances. For example, a child with autistism might continually swing a string of plastic beads, or spin endlessly on a tire swing.

SOME VARIATIONS

Asperger's syndrome is a milder form of autism. When classic autism and Asperger's syndrome are included with Pervasive Developmental Disorder, these illnesses comprise what is known as Autism Spectrum Disorder (ASD). Sometimes Rett Syndrome* is also included as an ASD. Attention Deficit Disorder (ADD) and Attention Deficit Hyperactivity Disorder (ADHD) are considered by many to be related to ASD because they appear to have similar causes and respond to

*Rett syndrome is a disorder of the nervous system that leads to developmental reversals, especially in areas of expressive language and hand use. It occurs almost exclusively in girls. Most cases are caused by a mutation in the MECP2 gene.

similar treatments. They may also coexist with autism. Some authors include both ADD and ADHD under the term ADHD.

DIFFERENT WAYS OF CARING FOR AUTISM

ASDs are not primarily psychiatric diseases, although some psychiatrists achieve good results in treating ASDs with mood altering medicines and various behavioral therapies. I believe the best current treatments for autism include medications to improve behavior; physical, occupational, and speech therapy; and biomedical interventions. All these therapies are indispensable for maximum treatment benefits. In a biomedical intervention, the first step is to determine what has gone wrong with an individual's normal body processes. The final steps in a biomedical intervention are to devise and provide an individualized treatment to correct and optimize an individual's bodily processes.

MY GOAL FOR BOOK

As a caregiver dedicated to treating autism, my hope is that this book helps both parents and caregivers of children with autism, as well as parents who wish to take measures to avoid having a child affected with autism.

HOW TO END AUTISM—LAST CHAPTER

This book ends by proposing a unique solution that has only been hinted at in other publications. I am very excited about defining and promoting this approach, and I sincerely hope and pray that this will open doors for the improvement and recovery of children with autism, doors that are currently frustratingly closed.

Let's get going!

Chapter One

Sink or Swim

The Problem

TAKE THE BALL AND RUN WITH IT

This chapter discusses a health-related problem that occurred in my family many years ago. My purpose in discussing these distressing events is to help the reader to understand that sometimes the only effective way to deal with perplexing health-related difficulties is to take matters into one's own hands. I propose that autism in America today is one of those situations that requires people, typically parents or parents-to-be, to take matters into their own hands. They must do this in order to protect their future children from the autism menace and to effectively nurture them, and do everything to heal any of their existing children who already suffer from it.

IS SHE OKAY?

Here is what happened in my family. One sunny summer afternoon, many years ago, my wife and I bicycled to an auto parts store. While I shopped my wife, Jill, waited outside for me. A few minutes later, the manager of the store paged me to tell me my wife had been in an accident in the parking lot. I hurried to the scene.

ODD BEHAVIOR

To my surprise I found Jill sitting on the ground leaning against the front bumper of a car. Her safety helmet was awkwardly cocked to the side and her bicycle was lying in front of her. She was crying, and when she saw me she asked me in a plaintive voice that was filled with anguish and distress, "What took you so long to come?" The driver of the car, an older man, stood beside her and said, "I tried to avoid her but she ran right into me." The man was telling the truth; Jill had run right into his car. My wife knew she was going to hit the car, but for some reason she just couldn't turn the handlebars to prevent it. She looked so pitiful there on the ground that I felt like crying too. Then the fire truck and the police came. Jill was checked out and the circumstances of the accident were reviewed. In a little while, she seemed well enough to be driven back home. It had been a painfully memorable afternoon.

GET TO THE ROOT OF THE PROBLEM

But this incident was not really an isolated one. Rather, it reflected a long-term health problem from which Jill was suffering. She had been having various symptoms that are related below for several years. These difficulties began shortly after we adopted Nikki, our first child. Our daughter was a poor sleeper and Jill's normal sleeping schedule was disrupted in caring for her. It was about this time that Jill's health began to deteriorate. We did not know the reason for her problem, but we suspected sleep deprivation or something else that occurred at about that time.

My wife became forgetful and began to do things that she had never done before, such as driving past places where she had appointments. In addition, her muscles ached severely. She also suffered from a crippling, energy-draining fatigue, and she had symptoms suggestive of low blood sugar. She was always freezing cold, even in the summertime. On the afternoon of the accident, she had forced herself to go on the bike ride, thinking that the exercise would help her to overcome her relentless lack of energy.

ALL WAS FINE IN THE PAST

Although Jill's health wasn't perfect before this time, it was good by ordinary standards. In fact, Jill had been employed for many years as a nurse and later as an Assistant Professor of Nursing with no health limitations. She had earned a master's degree and finished second in her class in the Pediatric Nurse Practitioner program at a respected Midwestern university before she retired to become a full-time mom.

NO, I WON'T ACCEPT THAT

At the time, I practiced medicine in an Internal Medicine clinic at a large hospital. I had been there for many years and my colleagues, whom we consulted, tried very hard to determine the nature of my wife's illness. All the standard tests for a condition like this --such as blood chemistry, brain waves and radiological studies-- failed to identify the cause of the problem. No one knew exactly what was wrong with Jill. They could only tell us that this seemed to be the beginning of a chronic, irreversible, deteriorative process and that we should try to enjoy the good times as long as we still had them.

The Solution

THE PROBLEM DISCOVERED

We were still young and our children quite young. We just couldn't accept this dismal prognosis, so we began to look into complementary and alternative medicine for answers. It was a matter of "sink or swim." We traveled all over the country in our quest for answers. Unfortunately, our medical insurance did not cover any of these expenses. The miles and the dollars climbed and climbed. However, the great news was that some clues and answers finally surfaced. It turned out that Jill suffered from an obscure problem called osteonecrosis of the jaw (1) as well as from chronic mercury intoxication. It appeared that her mercury-containing dental fillings were a major cause of the problem.

SOME WEAK, SOME STRONG

But why had this happened to Jill? Don't many people have dental amalgams containing mercury, even a mouthful of them, and not exhibit any of the symptoms from which my wife suffered? The answer is that each person's body chemistry is different. (2) In our investigations, we learned that the body has the ability to detoxify and excrete noxious substances, including mercury, and that the ability of individuals to eliminate such contaminants varies widely. In this light, depending on a particular person's level of noxious substances (called "toxic load") and their ability to excrete them, the problem can range from unnoticeable to severe.

MY WIFE HAD BEEN POISONED

In the case of harmful environmental substances, it's actually more hopeful to consider them as poisons rather than toxins. Clearing toxins evokes images of workers in white suits and masks attempting to clean a contaminated area, whereas eliminating poisons evokes the hope that an antidote might be available which can reverse the damage. With regard to chronic mercury poisoning the antidote is, first of all, to promptly remove any ongoing source of the contamination. The next step is to repair the body's biochemical routes and processes that are not adequately removing this harmful metal, allowing it to spread throughout the body. These biochemical routes and processes, known as detoxification pathways, largely reside in the liver. (3,4) In reality, both in Jill's case and in children with autism, some of these biochemical routes are blocked. Nearly all these blockages are inherited from a person's biological parents and grandparents and are abnormal from the start.

SOME CAN HANDLE IT, SOME CAN'T

Consequently, environmental chemicals and pharmaceutical drugs that can't be adequately processed and excreted become poisons to these individuals because of their genetic uniqueness. These "personal poisons" accumulate over time. They gradually, and sometimes suddenly, cause health problems --such as Jill's-- to occur. Perhaps the lack of sleep or something else that Jill's body had encountered at about the same time that our Nikki was adopted resulted in her body being unable to excrete her personal toxic burden, including mercury. Consequently, she experienced the symptoms related above. It is also known that the collective damage to the body is both multiplied by and manifested in a dwindling efficiency in all of the body's organs as a person ages. Deterioration in the structure and function of organs characterizes the aging process. In Jill's case, long-term stress, including sleep deprivation, in combination with her unique limitations in detoxification, may have caused enough organ deterioration and loss of function to impair her ability to rid her body of its toxic load and resulted in the symptoms she experienced.

THERE IS A REASON IT OCCURS

A person with autism suffers from health disorders similar to those Jill experienced. Research clearly reveals that autism is a disease of premature and accelerated aging of the body's organs, including the brain, through the mechanism of free radical damage. (5,6) Other autism-associated diseases present a similar picture. Injurious agents can also take the form of latent (covert) infections. Such a situation occurs when some viruses infect the brain and other organs. Chronic Lyme infection can do this also, and this disease may turn out to be the "sleeping giant" of autism. Disease develops when the body's immune surveillance system is too feeble to recognize and eliminate such microbial invaders. Sometimes the immune system becomes so over-stimulated that autoimmunity ("I am allergic to my own body tissue") or hyperimmunity develops. (7) The latter is an exaggerated response to a particular toxic metal, infection, or even to a required nutrient. Understanding how the body reacts to these types of dangerous invaders is important in understanding autism. Therefore, these topics will be covered in detail later on in this book (Chapter Six, "The Canary Children").

DOCTORS MUST LEARN MORE

Another similarity exists between Jill's medical experience and that of many children with autism. These children's parents frequently, almost universally, do not get clear answers and direction from conventional medical practitioners. Instead, they seem to encounter a lack of insight and understanding. These caregivers fail to recognize that autism is much more than a behavioral problem or a psychiatric diagnosis. ASDs encompass a complex set of abnormalities requiring much more than prescription drugs to improve behavior. Lots of treatment --such as speech, physical, and occupational therapies-- is needed, as well as supplements that are selected based on an understanding of the biochemistry that has gone amiss.

THE WEAK REQUIRE EXTRA CARE

Proper treatment for autism also includes an approach to effectively address the underlying problems of accumulating poisons and infections within an immature and developing organ system. In addition, these little individuals usually have inherited abnormalities in the detoxification pathways that were alluded to above. (8) Many parents of children with autism complain that traditional doctors do not have effective treatments and are unable to arrange for them. Others, who list themselves as autism practitioners, often claim that the answer lies uniquely in the programs they promote or in the supplements they sell. Experience has shown that this is rarely, if ever, the case.

I AM NOT GIVING UP

Thus, the situation that parents of children with autism face today is not unlike the situation my wife, Jill, and I faced many years ago: Either accept a dismal prognosis or work very hard, with drive and initiative, to find a solution. These parents must find and join forces with practitioners and organizations that have the experience and the ability to intervene in ways clinically proven to yield good results. It is, after all, a matter of "sink or swim".

Chapter Two

THE CUMULATIVE EFFECT

The Problem

The necessity of childhood vaccinations versus their safety is one of the most controversial issues we face today, perhaps even eclipsing a presidential election. In this chapter, I first intend to call the medical community to task and to exhort all its members to take a bold, active roll in a frontal attack on the disaster called autism.

Next, I will try to illustrate what makes some children less able than others to tolerate the currently recommended heavy vaccination load. I will then propose that this individual weakness is the causal link between immunizations and autism.

In **The Solution** section later in this chapter, I will suggest a workable approach to the vaccination dilemma. The chapter ends with a novel proposal to establish a new medical discipline.

Point number 7 in **The Solution** check list makes reference to what I believe is the fundamental "fix" that should effectively manage autism and even prevent its development. The last chapter of this book describes this approach.

This book was primarily written for parents. However, the autism problem belongs to all of us. And as the medical profession is part of the problem, so too must it be part of the solution. Along that line of thinking, I address my fellow physicians in the following short segment.

Something is wrong, very wrong. The medical community has fallen. It is fast losing the confidence of the American people. A new epidemic is the reason. It is a horrible situation for a young family. Some might even go so far as to call it a curse worse than death when a new baby boy or a young toddler is ruined for life because of autism. Instead of trying to meaningfully solve the problem by identifying and tackling what is wrong, the medical community seems to have "lost it".

Can you believe that, instead of "taking the bull by the horns" or "taking the ball and running with it" those who represent the medical community have become experts at finger pointing or have bailed out completely and allowed the vaccination companies to represent them and "call the shots", literally, over what they do? The whole issue is now a political football. It floods the news and talk shows, including stories of payoffs by vaccination companies.

This whole matter is enough to make one's blood boil!

If anyone wants to raise a voice in criticism of the above and state: “This man is himself a physician. Where is the science in what he writes?” I answer by asking: “Under what scientific discipline lies the commanding influence of the well-greased “for profit” vaccination machine on the practice of medicine? Who profits, who pays, and at what cost?”

WE MUST SERVE

I have personally been caring for children with autism for over ten years. My goal is to try to help as much as I can the overburdened parents who have to deal with this situation. Some of the families have suffered breakups. The father or mother can’t handle it, and the remaining spouse is left to care for the child alone. Short of a family breakup, I often see the burden of care for a child with autism fall disproportionately on one parent. I also witness how the ill child’s siblings suffer from a dearth of attention and love they too deserve.

It brings tears to your eyes to see a child who resembles other children in so many ways, and yet, one whom autism has made different in so many ways. Such a child has problems socializing, even just communicating; and how lamentable it is to try to make sense of what is going on in that beautiful, wonderfully intelligent brain, now caught up in repetitive acts and stifled by inflammatory damage.

This epic scourge of humanity must be stopped. And we doctors must do whatever is necessary to bring it to a quick end. We must act personally and not delegate decisions to suppliers or politicians. I appeal to all my fellow physicians to roll up their sleeves and get busy! A great need exists for our services. Therefore, we must serve!

HERE IS WHAT THEY THINK OF US

Putting my own passionate thoughts aside, I will now address the vaccination issue, and begin by acknowledging the controversy that surrounds the autism-vaccination issue. (9,10) Realizing that the vaccination controversy did not surface until autism became so prevalent, it now seems that any person with whom one speaks has a family member, a relative, or a friend who has a child with autism. Most of these people point their fingers at vaccinations and at the doctors who insist on giving them.

- They point out how much of a moneymaker vaccinations are for the companies who make them, and even for the doctors who prescribe them.

- They speak of financial contributions by vaccination suppliers to politicians.

- They observe parents who had normal, healthy children until they received the recommended vaccinations, followed by the child becoming severely ill and never being the same again.

- They speak of how they have reviewed all the websites and looked at the films on the You-Tube that show the before and after vaccination condition of a child, and which illustrate so convincingly the damage following the vaccination.

- They note how morally wrong it is for a child, in some cases even a baby, to be immunized against a sexually-transmitted disease, or how inappropriate it is for an infant to be given nine preservative-ridden immunizations, or 36 immunizations while still a toddler.

- They provide statistics that seem to prove that the medical community just blindly listens to the suppliers and then charges on with more --and even more vaccinations-- a "solve all" for all diseases.

- They wonder if there soon will be a vaccination for every type of illness and disease, such as cancer and diabetes. And why not? It seems the sky is the limit for the vaccination companies. Meanwhile, the rate of autism skyrockets!

LET'S AVOID THIS

Well, colleagues, have you heard enough? Is my point clear? A problem exists, even if you personally remain convinced autism does not develop in some individuals as the result of vaccinations. You must agree we physicians certainly have quite a wriggling mess on our hands. If we don't act soon, I seriously wonder if we are not leaving ourselves open to explicit public disdain. Why, we may eventually be dodging a barrage of well-aimed tomatoes!

LET'S SOLVE THE PROBLEM; WE CAN DO IT

Is what happens to us really important, compared with the agony of babies who become handicapped by autism for life? And what about the ordeal of the parents and society who must shoulder such an unremitting burden? I repeat my request: a plea for each and every one of us to "roll up our sleeves" and face the problem head-on. No more finger pointing! No more shifting this vital mission to vaccine suppliers and politicians! It is up to us, the medical profession, to get busy and solve this crisis that has already dragged on too long. We must show the public how much we really do care and that we are doing our best, given the circumstances with which we are dealing. What follows is my best shot at addressing this issue. My heartfelt hope is that it will help other physicians and parents to look this matter straight in the eye and without delay fix it, and fix it right.

NOT ALL ARE THE SAME INTERIORLY, EITHER

Chapter One introduced the concept that potentially injurious agents might be well tolerated by some individuals and poorly tolerated by others. This chapter applies the underlying mechanism for this person-to-person variability in tolerating vaccinations. This principle is called "biochemical individuality". This powerful concept was introduced by Roger Williams.(11) I believe that the "one size fits all" vaccination approach (which is basically what is occurring today in doctor's offices throughout our land) may be the wrong way to look at these childhood shots. I use the word "may" here to retain the skeptical reader. The error is in the failure to give proper consideration to each child's biochemical uniqueness.

SOME WEAK, OTHERS STRONG

Even if one considers administering childhood vaccinations to be as safe as drinking pure, fresh water, there are still medical situations, such as kidney failure and diabetes insipidus, wherein ingesting too much water can induce illness and even death. Whether the water will cure or kill boils down to the body's ability to handle a water load. And so it is with vaccinations. A particular child's ability to tolerate them is based on the child's biochemical makeup.

A WORKABLE APPROACH

I discussed this topic with the mother of a child with autism whose family physician regularly immunizes children in his practice. She told me he cares for thousands of children and is only aware of one or two cases of autism among his patients. Other doctors may make the same claim, but for the purposes of this book, I will focus on the experiences of two pediatricians for reasons set forth in the next paragraph. Isn't the lack of autism under these circumstances convincing evidence that vaccines don't cause autism?

RESULTS ARE IMPORTANT

This mother continued that this physician related to her that he believed the reason he sees little autism developing in his patients is because of the way in which he administers vaccinations to the children. This implies a safe way to administer vaccines to almost all children and that such a method is being followed in this practice. Because I was unable to speak directly with this doctor, I think it is best not to discuss his system, but to cover this methodology in a more general way by noting principles employed by experienced caregivers who have written on this topic. In an effort to validate this approach to the administration of vaccinations, I spoke with another pediatrician who offers a more relaxed immunization schedule to parents concerned about their children receiving too many shots too early in life. This doctor told me that he is unaware of autism developing in any of his pediatric patients. There may be an additional reason why this doctor is not seeing autism in his patients. This reason will be addressed later in this book.

BE OPEN TO CHANGE

The following is what I believe to be a very sensible approach to childhood vaccinations and it is a method that can be universally implemented today.

NOTE:

Before exploring the issue, I note that my practice involves treating children who have been diagnosed with autism. I do not offer childhood vaccinations, as my training and credentials are in internal medicine and nutrition. Therefore, I require my patients to also obtain medical care for their children from a family physician or with a pediatrician. In this way, the parents can also address the topic of vaccinations and specific vaccination schedules with that doctor, coupled with the general information presented here.

ABOUT THE DISEASE

Now I will briefly discuss "early onset autism" before returning to the topic of vaccinations. This form of autism occurs before, at, or shortly after birth. Some parents relate that their children did not look or act normal shortly after birth or when they took them home from the hospital. Other infants seem to deteriorate during their first year to the degree that something definitely seems to be wrong with the children. In fact, pictures of such afflicted children, taken at their first birthday parties, often reveal blank facial expressions and dull eyes.

TAKE OFF YOUR BLINDFOLD

A number of physicians who practice complementary or alternative medicine and treat patients with autism would certainly agree that parents frequently observe the development of full-blown autistic symptoms, especially in little boys, just before their second birthday. Autism that develops in this fashion is termed "late onset". Before developing autism, these children appeared to be completely normal, with timely developmental milestones. Not uncommonly, parents of these children relate that some of the vaccinations given to their children between 12 and 18 months of age were followed by hours of screaming and high fever, and by the gradual appearance of autistic symptoms, usually within weeks.

The association in time of autism developing in children, whose parents reported them experiencing a substantial vaccine reaction is such a common experience that, in the minds and hearts of many of these parents, it is difficult to believe these are just chance events.

DON'T BE BLIND TO THE FACTS

Two DVD's that discuss the vaccine controversy are available. (9,10). The reader could also get an idea of just how many adverse vaccine reactionsare reported by keying in something like "vaccines dangerous" into a good internet search engine. Vaccines, like the rest of the manipulated environment in which we live, must be continually scrutinized for their safety.

BE OBJECTIVE

Here is the other side of the coin: Vaccinations are nearly universally considered to be important health measures, and many children can apparently be safely immunized following current guidelines.

NO VACCINATIONS ARE NOT THE ANSWER, EITHER

It is also vitally important to learn the consequences of not vaccinating our children with one or more of the recommended vaccines. Those who favor mass immunizations worry that the large-scale refusal of parents to have their children vaccinated is creating a serious problem known as "loss of herd immunity." This means that, as the number of unvaccinated individuals continues to rise, a commensurate increase in infectious diseases in this susceptible fraction of the population can occur. Therefore, diseases such as polio, and *Haemophilus Influenzae* with their associated morbidity and even mortality --diseases nearly unheard of today-- may again become commonplace. Some health surveys are already beginning to report increases in communicable diseases that can be prevented by vaccination. It seems clear that, in some cases, vaccinations have been withheld for insufficient reasons, creating an incremental number of unprotected children. These children stand the chance of becoming seriously ill themselves and of transmitting their illnesses to those with whom they come into contact.

IN SUMMARY, SO FAR

All of this controversy brings us back to the ultimate questions:

> (1) Are there sufficient reasons to defer or limit vaccinations?
>
> (2) Is there a "safe" way to administer vaccines? This point refers to methods, such as those being practiced by the physicians mentioned above.

EXAMINING THE CUMULATIVE EFFECT

Let me begin with an analogy. Once, when I was riding in an outboard motor boat, a severe storm developed. The raging wind whipped up the water and soon a giant wave swept over the bow of the boat, dumping many gallons of water into it. This slowed the boat's progress but we were still able to continue toward the shelter of the shore at a reduced speed. Then another large wave hit the bow and still more water rolled in. We continued toward the shore but, burdened with more water, we moved even more slowly. When a third giant wave washed over the front of the boat it began to sink. Fortunately, by this time we could wade to safety. Although none of the three huge waves could have individually sunk the boat, the cumulative effect of all three waves did. Perhaps we might have remained afloat if we had been riding in a larger boat with its bow higher above the swelling waves.

SURVIVING THIS SEA

I believe this analogy explains what happens when a child in a weakened condition due to his or her unique biochemical make-up is exposed to a number of vaccinations at the same time. This child's biochemical machinery capacity renders him or her vulnerable to a large number of vaccinations given together for the following reason: each vaccine is meant to stimulate the immune system without overwhelming it, but not all immune systems function alike. Just as that small boat was sunk by the cumulative effect of three waves in a short time, a weakened immune system might not be able to tolerate multiple vaccinations given simultaneously and in quick succession.

A TIDAL WAVE FOR THE WEAK

Comparing this situation to a sinking boat is very relevant in view of the current practice of administering the measles-mumps-rubella vaccine in combination with the chicken pox, whooping cough, and hepatitis B vaccines. Alternatively, the first four vaccines are co-administered with the polyvalent pneumococcal vaccine and the vaccine against hepatitis A.(12) However, the manufacturer of the live, attenuated, measles-mumps-rubella vaccine indicates that given alone, it may suppress the immune system, resulting in a temporary reversion to negative (normal) of a positive tuberculin skin test. A positive skin test for tuberculosis is acquired through prior exposure to the tuberculosis bacterium (13).This vaccine-induced reversal from a positive to a negative TB skin test provides evidence that at least this part of the child's immune capacity has been compromised by vaccination against three viral diseases. One can only speculate how much more severe the effect would be when the usual larger number of vaccinations are given simultaneously.

A CHANGE FORTHE WORSE; LET'S CHANGE BACK

What happens when the above barrage of immunizations is administered to children who are ill-equipped to tolerate such a cumulative vaccination load? Does a connection exist between such a practice and the exponential rise in the incidence of autism to its current epidemic proportions? Contrast our current experience with the era when vaccinations were administered one at a time --not nine at one time-- and autism was rarely seen. In other words, is this practice, with all its health benefits to the population at large, its convenience, and even financial benefit to some --when looked at from the viewpoint of the individual person-- overwhelming the immune system of some children and resulting in autism and perhaps in ADHD as well?

NOT ONE DERANGEMENT, BUT MANY

Practitioners caring for children with autism, as well as parents, recognize that these children have alterations in their immunity ranging from underfunction, such as the susceptibility to many simultaneous infections, or to overactive immune situations, as multiple allergies and autoimmunity. Perhaps such immune impairments came first and autism is the consequence, not the cause of them. In addition, the ravages of autism inflict further damage on the child's already weakened immune system.

IDENTIFY THE WEAK AND BE EASY ON THEM

The point here is that, if some clinical clue of immune impairment exists, either in a particular child, in a sibling, or in relatives, living or dead, then this child may be "riding in a smaller boat." All of the foregoing are warning signs that this child may not be able to safely handle the oncoming immunization wave. As we cannot change the size of the boat, we will have to change the strength of the waves if we want to insure that this little person can enjoy safe passage through childhood. This means the immunization schedule needs moderation, such as spreading out the immunizations and returning to the practice of individual dosing.

THERE ARE ALWAYS RISKS

Adoption of this method might decrease the number of immunizations an individual receives and force some prioritization in their selection due to tailoring immunizations to the needs and tolerances of the individual child. An important counterpoint here is the risk of developing certain infectious diseases due to the omission of --or insufficient dosing of-- vaccines to prevent these very diseases, both in a particular child and in all those with whom this child is in contact.

THE ANSWER MAY BE A SIMPLE ONE

This proposal may meet with vigorous opposition from certain sectors and interests, but it also has health benefits, including, I believe, a lower incidence of autism. A country, as the U.S, possessing the logistics to put a man on the moon half a century ago, should certainly be able to implement the proposals made in this and upcoming chapters. Not all of them, I hasten to add, involve a watered-down vaccination schedule.

NOTE:

Next, we are going to present what many would deem a long list of precautions and warnings to be considered before administering a childhood vaccination. I acknowledge the dismay this discussion may create in the minds and hearts of those who are firmly convinced vaccinations are, by and large, safe. In addition, these sincere people may fear further dangerous erosion of herd immunity by large scale adherence to these warnings. I believe there are ways in which vaccinations can be safely given to most children. Later in this book, I will discuss a country where the incidence of autism is low, despite a rigorous immunization schedule. I will advocate adoption of a similar methodology. So please continue reading. And thank you for your forbearance.

IDENTIFY THE WEAK

My sources for the information that follows, in addition to my own experience gained in caring for children with autism, are physicians that are well versed in administering vaccinations to children, such as the two doctors who have written books on this topic and to whom I refer below. I also consulted the *Physicians Desk Reference* ®.

What familial clues should cause parents and physicians to exercise great caution before they subject a child to a rigid schedule of recommended immunizations, many of them combined? First of all, a family history of ASD, ADD, or ADHD should sound major alarms. Also, if the child has relatives who are suffering from diseases having immune features, such as rheumatoid arthritis, lupus and other collagen diseases, even type I diabetes, this should "raise a red flag."

LET'S DO OUR HOMEWORK FIRST

Any deteriorative disease of the nervous system, such as Alzheimer's, Parkinson's, multiple sclerosis, or amyotrophic lateral sclerosis (ALS, Lou Gehrig disease) is troubling, because autism itself results in the deterioration of both brain structure and function. Seizures in the individual, in the family, or a personal history of prior brain injury should also raise concern. These latter two conditions are listed in the warning category of the vaccine description in the *Physicians' Desk Reference* ® by the vaccine manufacturer. (13) Also, parallels have been drawn between autism, schizophrenia, and other behavioral disorders, such as obsessive compulsive disorder (OCD). A family history of any of these conditions needs to be taken into account in the vaccine decision making.

THE SICK NEED TIME TO RECOVER

Many temporary health problems also impair immunity. For example, if the body's immune system is already coping with an infection, or is in a state of fatigue or depletion from just having battled one, it is definitely weakened. I do not agree with those authorities who espouse the safety of vaccines, despite the presence of a mild fever, diarrhea, URI (upper respiratory infections), or other low grade febrile illnesses. I certainly feel that if the child is ill enough to keep home from school, then the immune system is probably significantly weakened and vaccines should not be administered under these circumstances.

THE INFANT IS NOT AN ADULT

One very natural situation of impaired immunity exists in the newborn. At this stage in life, the immune system is still underdeveloped in its ability to manufacture antibodies. Therefore, infants must depend on the passive transfer of antibodies in breast milk for their immunity against diseases. This being the case, one certainly could question the wisdom of administering the hepatitis B vaccine on the day of birth. Yet, this has been the modern day practice. Even infants at low risk for acquiring hepatitis B are typically immunized. Also, today many mothers choose not to breastfeed. These non-breastfed children are immunologically weaker, since they have not received the antibodies they would normally have been given in mother's milk.

THINK, STUDY, DELIBERATE BEFORE YOU ACT

There is no argument that the administration of multiple immunizations in close succession is a convenient and effective way of getting the schedule completed and of achieving herd immunity. But this practice fails to take into account the variation in individual immune systems, some of which might not safely tolerate such an immune (antigenic) load. We just don't fully understand how the many factors mentioned above can affect a child's immune system, and therefore the child's capacity to tolerate such vaccination practices. And we are only beginning to gain an understanding of what happens when many parents decide to universally defer or avoid all vaccinations.

PRECEDENT ESTABLISHED

A parallel to giving multiple vaccinations in children is the administration of multiple medications to elderly adults, another medically frail group. Pharmacists and physicians, especially those working with inpatients, have noted that when the number of concurrently administered prescription drugs increases, the chance of a medication interaction or drug-related adverse affect approaches 70 % (14). A physician who attends patients in a nursing home told me it was common to have patients admitted to him who are on nine medications.

A FLASHING WARNING SIGN

Polypharmacy, or the administration of a large number of medications to one patient, is unfortunately not limited to elderly patients in the hospital or in nursing homes. It is common in another vulnerable group which is at the other extreme of life, young children. Complications from treatment are more serious in children than they are in adults. Those with uncommon conditions have the highest cumulative medication dose exposure, and medications started in childhood for management of children with chronic conditions are often continued for decades. Infants admitted to children's hospitals may receive as many as 11 drugs concurrently.

This information appeared in a Medscape Education Clinical Brief authored by Kate Johnson. Ms. Johnson summarized a 2012 article by Freudtner and colleagues from the University of Pennsylvania School of Medicine and a related editorial by two physicians from Dartmouth Medical School that was published in a pediatric journal. This article validated earlier findings that acetaminophen was the most commonly prescribed medication to pediatric inpatients. Other drugs of concern in the Freudtner article were antibiotics and vaccines. This is such important material that it appears in its entirety in Appendix A.

IMPORTANT QUESTION

Where does all this foregoing information leave us? How can it be helpful to parents of children with autism and to future parents wishing to explore strategies to avoid autism and other adverse conditions in their children?

The Solution

A CHECKLIST

Reasonable approaches to immunizations have been set forth in excellently written publications about childhood vaccinations, such as the recently updated classic by Stephanie Cave, M.D.(15) and the book by Robert W. Sears, M.D. (16) In addition, Dr. Cave presented a protocol for childhood vaccinations in Alexandria, VA, in the Spring, 2007 national meeting sponsored by the Autism Research Institute. (17)

Using those guidelines and adding a few from other sources, parents or caregivers should consider the following points:

1) Is my child sick now or still in a weakened state from a recent illness? Vaccines shouldn't be given to ill children, such as those with fevers or colds, or if they are receiving antibiotics. Dr. Cabot also mentions this in her forward to this book.

2) A personal, or even a family history of a bad reaction to a vaccination or deterioration in health after a previous vaccination, should prompt the parents or caregivers to make a careful "risk vs. benefit" analysis. Ask these questions of yourself: "How important is it that my child receives protection against this particular disease at this time? How important is it to society that my child receives this vaccination now?"

3) Likewise, the knowledge of personal or family history of convulsions (seizures), deteriorative neurological diseases, or immune system disorders, such as those listed in the paragraph above entitled "LET'S DO OUR HOME WORK FIRST" should prompt a similar risk vs. benefit analysis.

4) Some authorities, such as those referenced above, recommend that vaccinations should be separated in time, i.e., not administered many at a time. Parents also have the option of delaying the first vaccination until the age of two years. Also, due to the many observations noted by parents, as well as by caregivers treating autism, of adverse experiences following combined measles, mumps, and rubella immunizations, these vaccines should

--if at all possible-- be given separately. This is very easy to say, but in practice may be very difficult to accomplish, since single-entity vaccines have recently not been available. And, there is the risk of contraction of an illness due to deferment of inoculation against it.

5) Parents should ask to examine the label on the vaccine bottle --even the box in which it came-- to ensure it doesn't contain thimerosal, a mercury-containing preservative used in multiple-dose vials where there is repeated needle entry.

On July 8, 1999, the U.S. Public Health Service declared its intention to "phase out" thimerosal from childhood vaccines because the recommended vaccination schedule exceeded the limits of mercury exposure. Today, most childhood vaccines are mercury-free, but the ultimate transition to zero is incomplete. For example, some flu vaccines given to children still contain thimerosal. (18)

6) Sometimes repeat immunizations, called "booster doses," aren't necessary. This is the case if protective titers (antibodies) against the infection that the immunization is formulated to prevent are already present in the blood. The child's blood can be tested for these titers. Consult with your pediatrician or family physician in the matter.

7) Several authorities suggest that doses of vitamins C and A, and the detoxifying antioxidant, glutathione (GSH), be given for two days prior to receiving vaccinations --See Dr. Cave's book on

childhood vaccinations referred to above for doses. (15) These are all ways to help support the liver and immune system during the stress imposed by a vaccination load. In Chapter Six, I focus on how critical it is to support the liver. You will see this applies not only to children, but to nursing mothers, and even to prospective mothers. In this final chapter, I establish the need for screening tests, especially those involving liver health. I will recommend these investigations be performed on infants before vaccination, as well as on mothers, and even on those contemplating motherhood

8) Parents should become familiar with the side effects of a particular vaccine and how to identify and report any adverse reaction which may occur. Keep a record of the vaccine manufacturer's name and the vaccine lot number.

9) Provide children with nutrient-rich diets and eliminate adverse environmental exposures, such as lead, asbestos, chemicals, pesticides, food additives, and over-processed food.

10) Parents should consider determining if their child harbors a significant toxic metal burden, such as lead, mercury, or arsenic that can impair the immune system. This can be done by consulting with a health care practitioner who is familiar with this procedure and who will send the specimen to a laboratory, such as Genova Diagnostics (Genova), Doctor's Data,Inc. (DD), or The Great Plains Laboratory (GPL). Contact information for these and other laboratories appears in the "Resources"

section at the end of this book. These facilities are equipped to detect the presence of even small amounts of toxic metals. Standard laboratories may fail to give proper attention to the presence of small amounts of toxic metals that are nevertheless harmful. This recommendation is especially relevant if the children themselves are known to have been exposed to toxic metals or if the family history is positive for the presence of such metals, such as lead intoxication that was acquired in the workplace.

11) The presence of colic or diarrhea, the failure to thrive, or the inability to gain weight can indicate long term immune impairment. In this event I advise that your practitioner investigate the health of your child's immune system before administering any vaccine containing live viruses.

12) Educate before you vaccinate. In addition to the above information consider visiting the National Vaccine Information Center's (NVIC) website for the viewpoint of parents who strongly feel their children were damaged by the vaccines they received.(19) Admittedly, this is a polarized group and their discussions certainly reflect their strong convictions. The disquieting question is: "Are these people correct in their allegations?"

LET'S GET SERIOUS ABOUT VACCINATIONS

Note that the above list was compiled to place the final decision regarding immunizations in the hands of the parents or caregivers. And I hope that such a decision will be made only after thoroughly discussing the pros and cons with a competent, informed, and unbiased heath care provider. Such decisions are not easy to make, and those made hastily may reap dire consequences. To facilitate your decision, you could carefully construct a risk vs. benefit analysis.

THINK, STUDY, DELIBERATE BEFORE ACTING

Conceivably, some risk factors would be present in practically every case if one tries to apply a comprehensive list of all possible contraindications. Therefore, it becomes a matter of relative risk. As the number of "red flags" increases, the decision to vaccinate becomes increasingly more difficult and perhaps downright wrong. But reason must rule. For example, following current recommended schedules and guidelines, one could seriously question the wisdom of immunizing a child whose sibling has autism, or one who has a personal history of seizures and multiple allergies. It would also seem unwise to vaccinate a child who had prior severe adverse reactions to multiple vaccinations, and whose family history includes rheumatoid arthritis, multiple sclerosis, or Alzheimer's disease.

GREEN LIGHT

However, based on our current knowledge of the safety of vaccines for most persons, it would seem reasonable to vaccinate a perfectly healthy child whose family history is negative for the illnesses and conditions noted above. Upcoming sections of this book that address the importance of the liver health will, I believe, explain my reasons for using the qualifying term " seem".

PREFERED WAY

Also, to decrease the number of added chemical preservatives and other adulterants, pending their availability, single entity vaccines dispensed from single dose vials. Preservative-free vials are by far the most desirable for some children.

HUMAN NATURE POPS UP ITS HEAD

I acknowledge that some topics and references in this chapter are highly emotionally charged material. In such cases, the reader must make the effort to glean fact from fervor. The answer to why an author who believes in the importance of vaccinations would even include such material lies in his earnest effort to uncover the bare truth of this grave matter. Unfortunately, review of the forces tugging from all directions on the immunization ring also reveals some vectors of science, medicine, and industry that are lamentably tainted by inflexibility and arrogance, as well as the by the enticement of monetary gain, all to the detriment of our children.

THE GOAL TO SHOOT FOR

I believe the pure solution to the vaccination problem must flow through a gate of enlightened humility --held open by a generosity that surrenders every tenet and talent-- in order to find the formula that will end autism once and for all.

NOTHING SPEAKS LIKE RESULTS

An interesting experimental "study", albeit an unplanned one, is occurring in the United States and Canada. This circumstance provides an answer of sorts to the question of the incidence of autism in largely unvaccinated population groups, such as home-schoolers or the Amish. The wholesome, natural lifestyle of the Amish undoubtedly confers protection against the diseases against which we immunize. And, as we shall see later in this book, lifestyle may be an important --perhaps the most important-- determinant in the prevention of autism. Also, from speaking with Amish people, I have learned that they often defer the first vaccination until the child is two years old. In many cases, immunizations are never given.

BE SCIENTIFIC: LOOK AT THESE FACTS

In 2005 Dan Olmsted began looking for autism in major

Amish population centers. He notes that only a few cases of autism exist in the United States with a total population of almost two hundred thousand Amish, largely concentrated in three states. Using the then current estimated nation-wide prevalence of autism of 1 in 150 live births, Olmsted expected to find about 1,000 cases among the Amish. However, he was able to identify only a handful of cases, less than twenty, yielding a rate of one in ten thousand --about one hundred times less than the current best estimates. Olmsted relates that, in the fifteen thousand Amish children living near Middlefield, Ohio the director of a Clinic for Special Needs Children in Ohio, Dr. Heng Wang, is aware of only one case of autism. (20)

COULD SOMEONE BE INFLUENCING CONGRESS?

A similar situation exists in Lancaster County, Pennsylvania. A physician practicing there, Frank Noonan, who has cared for thousands of Amish patients spanning twenty five years, said with regard to autism, "We're right in the heart of Amish country and seeing none, and that's just the way it is." Olmsted teamed up with Mark Blaxhill who is the father of a child with autism. These authors relate in their book on autism that the former director of the CDC in Atlanta, Dr. Julie Gerberdling, has said that studies of autism rates in never-vaccinated American children "could be done and should be done". However, Congress has repeatedly failed to move on a bill requiring the federal government to conduct such a study. (20)

VACCINATIONS ARE JUST PART OF THE PROBLEM

The cumulative-dose principle addressed in this chapter applies not only to multiple simultaneous vaccinations, but also to the additive, or even multiplicative damage to the human body caused by concurrent exposure to numerous environmental poisons. This is the principle of the "total toxic load." Because of our environment becoming so menacingly contaminated, Chapter Six is dedicated to discussing this disaster of our industrialized world and what can be done by a family, parent, or caregiver to effectively deal with it.

LONG-TERM SOLUTION

Reflecting on the above list and all the considerations and factors --including the fact that a wrong decision and action may result in a human being growing up with severe mental and physical problems-- the need for change should be obvious. The medical community needs to create a new discipline that specializes in the administration of vaccinations and the necessary weighing of individual data and decision-making prior to immunizing.

A DOCTOR WITH AN IMPORTANT RESPONSIBILITY

We propose that a separate doctor should be in charge of giving all vaccinations to children. This physician would spend all the time necessary to prevent permanent damage to any child from wrongful or error-ridden administration of childhood vaccinations.

MY RECOMMENDATION

I believe this type of specialization is more than justified, and I urge that the medical schools should begin the classes and certification programs immediately.

MEDICALLY, IT JUST MAKES SENSE

I believe creation of such a discipline is the long-term solution to the problem. In addition, it will unburden pediatricians who have enough to learn and study on their own specialty.

FINANCIALLY, IT JUST MAKES SENSE

From a social and economic standpoint, it is more than justified. The burden to society, the social security system, and other governmental agencies for each child with autism is said to be in the millions of dollars.

LET'S DO WHAT IS RIGHT FOR THE RIGHT REASON

But far more importantly, we live in America and are supposed to be people who value freedom. All our citizens deserve the best care we can provide. This includes the defenseless baby in the mother's arms.

COMING UP NEXT

In the next chapter I explore one of the principal problems existing in autism. This problem is individualized and unique. It has far-reaching consequences, including adverse effects on the brain. And I will address how it can be diagnosed and managed. This problem lies within the gastrointestinal tract.

Chapter Three

The Enemy Within

The Problem

SUFFERING CHILDREN

Most children with ASDs suffer from gastrointestinal (G-I) disorders. I can conservatively state that at least 75% of the children that I have treated suffer from such problems. In fact, I have rarely found a child with ASD's who did not have some type of G-I problem. Some of these problems were constipation, in a few cases even fecal impaction, abdominal pain, gaseousness, diarrhea, and gastroesophageal reflux. The clue to abdominal pain in a non-verbal child is frequently when the child tries to relieve the pain by putting pressure on the abdomen while leaning over a piece of furniture.

SOME RELIEF

I have found that addressing abnormalities in the G-I tract is the one intervention that brings the greatest improvement in children with ASDs. This type of intervention begins with the elimination of gluten (found in foods containing or made from wheat, rye, barley and sometimes oats), and often casein-containing-foods (i.e. dairy, as milk, cheese, and all products made from them). Not uncommonly, removal of certain sugars, carbohydrates, and starches is often initially required.

THE EXPERTS HAVE SPOKEN

Recently, a group of respected pediatric gastroenterologists, all of whom were experienced in treating children with autism, wrote a consensus report and an article with their recommendations on how to manage G-I problems in children with ASDs. This information was published as two supplemental articles. (21,22) The articles are important because they were published in a mainstream medical journal, and they clearly document that G-I problems in autism are common and require special attention. Some of the contributing authors were very fervent in stressing the importance of the gut in treating autism. Many alternative and complementary caregivers by and large have long believed that autism is largely a below-the-diaphragm disease.

NOT JUST A G.I. PROBLEM

A major point of the report and article was that the G-I disorders in children with autism could cause them to suffer serious behavioral problems, such as recalcitrant stubbornness, self-injury, and aggression. Additional clues to a malfunctioning gut include sleeping disorders and even metabolic diseases that affect energy and neurologic sensory processing. In layman's terms, this means that G-I disorders can adversely affect how the brain takes in and sorts out messages from the five senses. My experience in treating children with autism bears out what the report and article claim, namely, that G-I disorders can cause many problems for these children. Such illnesses can also include celiac disease and long term G-I infections.

HERE IS WHAT WE WILL DISCUSS NOW

The overall goal of this book is to arrive at a solution for autism, its prevention, and its management and care. To increase this understanding, let us now examine what can go wrong in the G-I tract of children with autism and make an attempt to explain why these little individuals are particularly susceptible to G-I problems. I will also discuss the purpose and scope of some special diagnostic tests that can complement a thorough history and physical examination of the child and direct caregivers to tests and investigations that are often covered by insurance plans and can be very helpful in understanding autism.

A WHOLE ARMY EXISTS WITHIN US

In order to learn about "the enemy within" we must familiarize ourselves with two concepts. The first is called "dysbiosis." We all harbor living creatures in our G-I tracts from our mouths to our rectums. Some of them grow in our small intestine, an organ that specializes in absorbing the food we eat. The normal presence of these organisms enables the processes of food digestion and absorption to occur. We must appreciate that our health depends on what is living in our gut. These inhabitants, or flora, include bacteria, viruses, fungal agents, such as yeasts, and even parasites. The foregoing list makes it clear that both beneficial and unwanted organisms can reside in our G-I tract. An example of a beneficial organism is some *Bifidiobacteria* species. Examples of undesirable organisms are parasites and the presence of yeasts, such as *Candida,* when the latter is present in abnormally large numbers. Dysbiosis is a scientific term that simply means our intestines are harboring too many harmful organisms and too few of the good kind.

HOW DYSBIOSIS CAN DEVELOP IN A NEWBORN

G-I problems can occur at any time in life. However, my experience and reading brings to light the likelihood that these problems will seriously affect the physical and emotional well being of the individual throughout one's life, whether they begin during intrauterine life or within hours after birth.

A DELICATE SITUATION

Two factors interplay here. The first is the health of the mother during her pregnancy. Maternal health is addressed in Chapter Six and includes any adverse condition or illness that an expectant mom may be harboring in her body that could affect the normal development of the human being growing inside of her. The second is the birth itself. In a normal vaginal birth and subsequent breastfeeding of the baby, transfer of healthy organisms from the mother's intestinal tract to the child's intestinal tract occurs. This is part of a process is referred to in terms such as "fetal microbial imprinting". (23) Organisms, such as bacteria, that can only be seen through a microscope, are called microbes. This vaginal transfer of healthy organisms does not occur during a caesarian birth and it is impossible to achieve on formula food. Often, the recovery from a caesarian operation and the preference of the mother to rest undisturbed after even a vaginal delivery thwarts normal breast-feeding. The natural act of breastfeeding is the most important means of delivering healthy intestinal tract organisms from the mother to the child.

NATURE HAS ITS WAY

I now present an important, unknown (at least to us) matter that we learned from raising sheep. For the first few hours after breast milk begins to flow, it is largely comprised of a nearly magic yellowish material called colostrum. This occurs in the first milk of both humans and animals, and it is critical for the health of the baby or the newborn animal to receive it. I am also a shepherd, as you will learn later in the book, and raising animals provided us with a vital learning experience. We did not realize the importance of colostrum until our ewes (female sheep) delivered their baby lambs. We found that the lambs would die if they did not receive colostrum in the first 45 minutes of life. Having had this experience, it is understandable that the well-being of newborn human beings may similarly depend on the provision of colostrum available in mother's first milk.

HOW THE PROBLEM MAY BEGIN

A prematurely born child may be taken to the neonatal intensive care unit (NICU) where breast-feeding is more complicated, though not impossible. Here both antibiotics and corticosteroids --derivatives of the adrenal hormone cortisone-- are frequently administered. Such medications --albeit well-intended, often necessary, and sometimes even life saving-- nevertheless disrupt the normal microbial imprinting process in the baby's intestine. The care and medications provided in the NICU set the stage for inoculation of his or her intestine with a completely new and foreign set of organisms that are not suited to this time of life, and perhaps not to any time of life.(23)

A CHANGE FOR THE BETTER

In the NICU setting, the process of populating the baby's G-I tract is a chance event. The newborn's intestinal tract is sterile. No organisms are growing there, yet. Therefore, the first organisms to enter the child's intestinal tract in NICU, rather than being passed on from the mother, are picked up from the NICU environment including whatever organisms may be growing on the skin or even in the G-I tracts of hospital employees who have some contact with the NICU. (23) Healthful organisms (called probiotics) can be administered in this setting. I hope that this will become a universal part of NICU management.

NOT A GOOD START

The administration of antibiotics and corticosteroids in NICU creates conditions in the infant's G-I tract that allow a stubborn yeast colonization (as with *Candida*) to gain a foothold, perhaps even a lifelong entrenchment. In summary, in the NICU the baby's gastrointestinal tract is greatly predisposed to colonization with some undesirable organisms, rather than being populated with healthy ones. This situation is called dysbiosis. By the way, dysbiosis not only refers to infants' gastrointestinal tracts being infected with undesirable organisms rather than with healthy ones, but can develop at any time in life in the gastrointestinal tract. In fact, it also develops in some infants who were never admitted to the NICU.

WE ARE ALL IN THE SAME BOAT

Just like in the NICU setting, administrating antibiotics and/or steroids to young and old alike is frequently the initiating event allowing undesirable, rather than healthy organisms, to populate the intestinal tract. Antibiotics can have the side effect of eliminating healthy organisms in the intestinal tract, allowing its repopulation by non-healthy organisms. These undesirable "bugs" have a greater chance of gaining a foothold if some preexisting G-I mucosal damage, for example, from gluten or some milk, soy, or corn product is present.

WE'VE HEARD THIS BEFORE

Although vaginal delivery helps prevent dysbiosis from developing in a baby, the most protective measure against it, by far, is breastfeeding. Breastfeeding should be continued for months, or better still, for years. This is because the mother's milk is rich in protective antibodies and in desired organisms that the infant's G-I tract needs for normal growth and development, as well as for events which occur in the baby's body overall. The beneficial organisms are transported to the breast milk from the mother's G-I tract via the bloodstream by a special form of white blood cells called macrophages. Breastfeeding is nature's optimal means of nurturing, for it provides not only the desired flora, but also the helpful antibodies and other natural substances the baby so critically needs. Breast milk provides them in a form that is best digested and absorbed by the infant's G-I tract.

THE GOOD OUTWEIGHS THE BAD, BY FAR

Breastfeeding also raises the level of beneficial hormones (oxytocin and secretin) in both mother and child, while delaying or completely eliminating the introduction of synthetic formula feedings or exposure to other than human milk. Based on the experience of many physicians and patients, the early introduction of a soy-based formula or of cow's milk to an infant can often prove to be detrimental to that infant's health. These unnatural replacements for breast milk by soy-based formulas or cow's milk are unhealthy because they cannot be properly digested and utilized at this time of life. Substitutes for mother's milk do not provide many of the vital substances the baby requires that the mother provides from her G-I tract, liver, immune system, and her reservoir of vitamins and minerals in their natural forms. This is a major shortcoming of milk substitutes.

THE HYGEINE HYPOTHESIS

New Research from Harvard Medical School offers supporting evidence for the theory that reduced exposure to microbes during childhood increases susceptibility to certain diseases later by failing to promote natural development of the immune system. The scientists discovered that germ-free mice raised in sterile conditions accumulated more of a type of white blood cells called invariant natural killer T (iNKT) cells in their colon and lungs compared with mice raised in non-sterile conditions. These same kind of white cells are thought to have a role in ulcerative colitis and asthma in humans.(24)

TIMING IS ALL-IMPORTANT

Colonizing the germ-free mice with conventional bacteria prevented colitis and asthma sensitivity and kept iNKT cells from accumulating, but only if the mice were exposed to the bacteria right after birth.(24)

TAKE ME HOME

The reporter of this information accompanied it with a picture of a young girl petting a farm animal, apparently to indicate that the girl might thereby acquire some beneficial organisms from the animal. The good organisms that are acquired early in life, such as may be occurring in this picture, are sometimes referred to as "Old Friends".(25)

CLEAN, BUT NOT TOO CLEAN

Attempts to over-protect children from environmental events as the usual childhood diseases may have its disadvantages. Families with fewer children provide lesser opportunity for cross-infections of childhood viral illnesses at a time in life when they usually pursue a benign course. In addition, use of antibiotics disrupts the healthy microbiota, in other words, normal intestinal flora, and opens up opportunities for potential pathogens to replace them. Nature has a way to counter this. It is the exchange of beneficial organisms between farm animals and humans who are in contact with them. This is only one of the many advantages that can accrue to a family that keeps some of the smaller species of such animals. I will address the many benefits of this practice in more detail in Chapter Five.

A PARTING LOOK AT DYSBIOSIS

When antibiotics are administered to persons of any age, a reduction in healthful microbiota occurs, and so the cells of the mucosal surface of the colon, for example, those that line the inner wall of that part of the G-I tract, become inflamed. Inflammation is a term used to describe the development of warmth, redness, swelling, and pain. A lesser number of healthful microbiota results in a diminished production of short-chain fatty acids (SCFA), of which butyrate is an example. The role of butyrates and other SCFA is to nurture these cells in the colon. Thus, as a result of the lack of sufficient healthful flora, these intestinal cells become both inflamed and malnourished.

Should enzyme production falter due to inflamed and malnourished intestinal lining cells, normal digestion will decrease. This is because the role of enzymes in the G-I tract is to convert food particles into absorbable forms. Diminished enzymatic digestion results in an accumulation of rich, unabsorbed nutrients in the G-I tract. Then abnormal microflora, that we could call opportunistic squatters, enjoy an excess of nutrients on which to feed and thrive. As noted above, the expansion of abnormal microflora at the expense of healthy organisms is called dysbiosis, and the harmful biochemicals they produce inflict further damage on the mucosal cells (26,27,28, 29).

LET'S SWITCH SUBJECTS

The last few paragraphs have introduced a number of new facts and concepts to most readers. How dysbiosis originates is very important for readers to understand. Many diseases can cause dysbiosis if the intestinal conditions of the individual are favorable for its development. The next section of the text describes the damage that dysbiosis can inflict on the body organs of persons of any age.

WHAT IS BIOFILM?

Gut microbiota stimulate intestinal lining cells to produce mucus, a sticky biological substance. Biofilm, on the other hand, is a matrix produced by microbes in which they can reside. Mucus is not part of G-I biofilm, although biofilm can be located wtihin mucus, on the mucus layer, or on the intestinal mucosal lining itself. It is made by virtually all bacterial and single-celled fungi. Biofilms are highly-ordered, often multi-species, protected communities of micro-organisms within which the various co-adhesed organisms cooperate, communicate, and in other fashions regulate each other's mode of existence and survival. Specific components of the biofilm interact with and can neutralize antibiotics. Pathogenic (disease-producing) microbes have been shown to preferentially increase the thickness of the biofilm matrix layer when exposed to antibiotics. Biofilm formation is now recognized as the major reason for antibiotic resistance by pathogenic bacterial and fungal strains.(28) It is by no means confined to the G-I tract and is thought to underlie infections throughout the body ranging from dental caries to those on implanted medical devices, such as prosthetic joints.

We can look upon biofilm as a biological apartment building inside the gut. It is neither good nor bad, as the microbes producing it can be healthful or potentially pathogenic ones. What makes biofilm undesirable is what makes a tenement building undesirable: the treacherous tenants living there.

HOPEFUL NEWS

Commercially available products to control biofilm involve the use of antibiotics as well as enzymes that digest this microbe-made matrix. Metal-binding agents in natural or synthetic form are added, as some bacterial pathogens thrive on, for example, iron. Removal of iron by these chelating agents hampers their growth. Anti-biofilm agents are administered apart from food to facilitate pathogenic organism destruction as biofilm is degraded. Prebiotics and probiotics also have their treatment role. *Lactobacillus* species demonstrates a significant ability to inhibit biofilms of undesirable species.(27,28)

THANKS, COLLEAGUES

Dr. Anju Usman has initially investigated the role biofilm plays in the intestinal tracts of children with autism. Dr. Stephen Olmstead has kindly reviewed the material presented in this chapter and suggested many helpful modifications.

ALERT

On his website*, Dr. Mercola has recently called attention to the deleterious contribution to biofilm formation that appears to result from the addition of a flowing agent, magnesium stearate, by drug and supplement manufacturers to facilitate passage of their product through processing machinery and capsular filling. The information provided on this website notes that, in addition to this reported deleterious effect on biofilm formation, magnesium stearate provides no nutritional value. The stearic acid component of magnesium stearate has been experimentally shown to decrease formation of T cells, natural killer cells, thus impairing immune function. In our family we now try to find powdered or liquid forms of supplements to avoid this problem.

*articles.mercola.com/sites/.../whole-food-supplement-dangers

THE DOMINO EFFECT

When the G-I tract is weakened, the G-I immunity in the form of the gastrointestinal associated lymphoid tissue (G.A.L.T.) and mucosal associated lymphoid tissue (M.A.L.T.) undergo marked anatomic and functional change. These adaptations can include intense over stimulation and lead to lymphoid nodular hypertrophy (L.N.H.) that takes the form of numerous large bumps on the inner intestinal wall.

This research was initially done by Dr. Andrew Wakefield who came under broad attack for his work. However, the presence of LNH in the intestines of children with autism has recently been confirmed by other investigators.(30) These bumps are made up of lymphocytes, a form of white blood cells that can travel in the bloodstream or can reside permanently at one location in the body. In the condition called LNH, lymphocytes accumulate in the intestinal wall.

It's my understanding that lymphocytes in the wall of the G-I tract (and in other mucosal surfaces throughout the body, such as the respiratory tract) may either overproduce, or worse, underproduce the important protective immunoglobulin called secretory IgA. This immunoglobulin can be measured in a stool specimen if it is sent to Doctors Data. A high intestinal IgA value indicates that the body's immune system is in a heated battle with the dysbiosis. A low IgA value indicates the depletion of this important defense mechanism.

RESOURCES

For the reader interested in learning more about the important role that gut flora plays in the life of the newborn and very young child, I recommend some of the material referenced above that is very accessible on the internet. (23,25,27)

ANOTHER WAY THE PROBLEM CAN BEGIN

Although the following finding is oftentimes not grasped and accepted, it is important to describe how the presence of heavy metals, such as mercury, arsenic, and lead in the body, can also lead to dysbiosis. By their presence within the G-I tract, these metals are suspected to impair the immune system's ability to suppress the growth of pathogenic organisms, frequently resulting in the increase in large numbers of yeast and harmful bacteria. (31) Dr. Stephanie Cave, who has cared for more than 10,000 children with autism, calls attention in her presentations to the see-saw battle that can exist in the gut between control of dysbiosis and its rampant flaring. This latter situation occurs when heavy metals enter the gut through the bile in the process of their removal from body stores during special measures to promote their clearance. She notes this effect is sometimes so pronounced that the practitioner must discontinue such procedures and redirect attention to the dysbiosis.(32) The management of dysbiosis will be addressed in the Solution part of this chapter.

THE PROBLEM WORSENS

In addition to grasping the significance of dysbiosis, understanding "The Enemy Within" also requires the presentation of a second concept: the loss of the normal barrier function of the intestinal mucosa that occurs due to inflammation. The gut lining reacts violently when exposed to something it regards as toxic, for example, gluten. It also reacts with similar force when the intestinal contents become infected with undesirable, and sometimes pathogenic flora, such as abnormally large amounts of the bacterial species *Clostridium* or the yeast, *Candida*. As I will note in **The Solution** section of this chapter, *Clostridium* may constitute up to 30% of the stool microbiota. Therefore, the report of *Clostridium* on stool examination may not in itself indicate the presence of a pathogenic organism. The word pathogenic means capable of causing disease.

Recall that in dysbiosis, populations of healthy bacteria, such as *Bifidobacteria,* and some beneficial *E. coli* strains, dwindle. These "good bugs" get crowded out by the "bad ones". The small intestine, which normally contains many less organisms than are present in the colon, becomes overpopulated with microbes, although this overgrowth is not necessarily of pathogens. Usually, in fact, it is an overgrowth of normal intestinal organisms. (33) As previously mentioned, the use of antibiotics promotes the growth of yeast, as do high levels of hormones, including sex hormones and adrenal cortisol. These hormones may originate inside the body, or they may be introduced into the body from prescription medications containing their synthetic forms.

WHAT IS LEAKY GUT?

Inflammation of the gut lining causes a breakdown not only of its anatomic cellular integrity, the intactness of the cell itself, but also of the intercellular (between the cells) glue that holds the cells together. The individual cells, the building blocks lined up side by side which form the inside surface of our intestinal wall, figuratively speaking, lose their "water proofing". They become porous. Thus, these intestinal lining or "mucosal" cells lose their shoulder-to-shoulder tightness such that substances can squeeze between them and gain entry to the body. Such a barrier breakdown results in abnormally large passageways developing both through and inbetween these mucosal lining cells. Huge molecules of undigested food and other substances, in a form that is both unfamiliar and unacceptable to the body, that ordinarily would have remained as intestinal contents, are now able to seep through these abnormal openings and enter the bloodstream. When this occurs, the body mounts a reaction against these foreign materials. The presence of these undigested substances elicits an immune response because they are in a place where they do not belong.

Immune responses include symptoms of all sorts, such as reactions to certain foods, rashes, eczema, sleep disorders, fibromyalgia, migraines, and arthritis.(34) The body's reaction to the presence of these foreign substances can also be manifested by the obstreperous behavior all too familiar to the parents of children with autism. It appears that the brain is registering its own kind of allergic reaction, not by developing a rash or a wheeze, but through a very evident worsening of behavior.

The open gastrointestinal barrier with increased intestinal permeability caused by the inflammation of the gut in response to something it regards as toxic is what is known as a "leaky gut". The body's response to this inward-directed G-I leakiness are all the symptoms we have just mentioned.

ME TOO

If you have any of the symptoms noted above, even though you may not suffer with autism, the cause may be that you are also harboring a leaky gut. I find this to be common, even in my adult patients, and one that frequently responds to the clinical management that is to follow.

MORE RESOURCES

A treatment of this topic that is short and well worth reading in an article entitled "Surprises from Celiac Disease" by Dr. Alessio Fasano. (35)

MORE PROBLEMS TO SOLVE

Recent research discloses that the body can also react

systemically, that is, “body-wide”, to an irritating food or a pathogenic organism present in the G-I tract, even in the presence of an intact, intestinal mucosa. The irritation stimulates gut immune cells to produce locally active chemical messengers, called cytokines, that inflame the inside of the small intestine. These cytokines also can be absorbed and cause a great deal of mischief similar to that caused by large, foreign molecules themselves passing through abnormal channels between and through damaged cells.(36)

ANOTHER PIECE OF THE PUZZLE

Individuals with leaky gut suffer from an additional problem. Potent toxins, generated by accumulating hostile organisms make their way into the bloodstream. Such blood-borne toxins can reach the brain where they engender behavioral havoc. Such emotional outbursts or meltdowns are encountered with some subtypes of *Clostridium* bacteria, and probably with a number of other unwelcome gut inhabitants as well. Research has shown that certain subtypes of *Clostridium* are present in children with autism.

IN SUMMARY

Intestinal dysbiosis and a leaky gut are important factors in what goes wrong with the G-I tract in an individual affected by autism. In addition, a clinical review published several years ago linked irritable bowel syndrome, a commonly encountered disorder affecting all age groups, to bacterial overgrowth in the small intestine. (33)

The Solution

RECOMMENDED DIAGNOSTIC TESTS

A disease must be properly diagnosed before it can be correctly managed. This is particularly true of diseases affecting the G-I tract. Unfortunately, standard laboratory tests do not always identify the presence of pathogenic organisms in the G-I tract. However, some non-standard tests do identify these pathogenic organisms. A number of alternative and traditional practitioners are aware of these investigations. Dr. Stephanie Cave has stated that one of these studies, the organic acids analysis, is for her the most valuable diagnostic test.(32) The organic acids analysis provides a wealth of information. Frequently, this is the first laboratory investigation that I request. Unfortunately, it is not always covered by standard health insurance, but it may be reimbursed through a health spending account.

A simple morning urine specimen is all that is required. The test provides information about an individual's cellular metabolism, the adequacy of their key vitamins, the chemistry of their neurotransmitters, and also indicates the presence of some environmental toxins in their bodies. The term "cellular metabolism", also called intermediary metabolism, refers to the individual's biochemical Krebs cycle, a magnificent mechanism wherein proteins, carbohydrates and fats all are transformed into forerunner compounds (called precursors) of ATP, the body's energy molecule. ATP is the fuel for nearly all body processes, such as muscle contraction and digestion.

The neurotransmitters mentioned above have the function of carrying on vital informational cross-talk or communication within the brain.

VERY REVEALING

Remarkably, the organic acids analysis also can indicate the presence of G-I problems. It can detect certain biochemicals made during the intestinal growth of some pathogenic bacteria and fungi, such as disease-producing *Clostridium* strains and yeast. These products of microbial metabolism end up in the urine after first having been absorbed from the G-I tract into the bloodstream and then filtered into the urine by the kidneys. In this fashion the organic acids test can denote the presence of disease-causing organisms in the G-I tract. This feature makes it a very valuable diagnostic test. It is especially useful because stool samples sent to the laboratory for microscopic analysis and for culture (meaning growth under laboratory conditions) may not reveal the presence of pathogens.

The reason for this is that many intestinal pathogenic organisms are anaerobic, meaning that they only grow in low-oxygen environments. Thus, even though these oxygen-shunning organisms were reproducing in the anaerobic environment of the small bowel, they would not be detected by culturing the stool in the standard manner. As soon as the stool passes outside of the body, it enters an oxygen-rich atmosphere and conditions change to what is termed aerobic. Therefore, these anaerobic bacteria die when they are exposed to atmospheric oxygen. But the chemical substances they make while they are growing in the body are not so sensitive to the atmosphere. They can be measured in the urine sample after they have been absorbed into the body through the G-I mucosa and filtered out of the body by the kidneys.

A number of laboratories offer the organic acids analysis, including the Great Plains Laboratory, Genova Diagnostics and the Metametrix Clinical Lab.

STOOL TESTING

I also frequently request the test that examines the stool itself. Culturing the stool in the special laboratories noted below and requesting they examine it directly under the microscope often reveals the presence of pathogens not picked up by the organic acids analysis and is the method of choice for identifying a number of the many species of G-I organisms. The microscopic examination can detect organisms in the stool that may have died during transport to the laboratory and therefore are no longer culturable. Thus, the "ghost forms" of some yeast can be visible on microscopic exam.

However, if the pathogens cannot be grown in the laboratory, they cannot be tested for their sensitivity to antimicrobial agents, so the microscopic presence of dead organisms isn't as useful as the culturing of live ones. The organic acid test also suffers from this shortcoming. I send my patients' stool specimens to Genova or to Doctors Data (DD) for analysis, and this stool analysis can also be ordered through the Great Plains Laboratory. These laboratories are listed on page 189.

CLOSTRIDIUM TESTING

Dr. David Quigg of DD Laboratory informed me that his company offers a procedure to study *Clostridim* more intensively. This technology capitalizes on the incredible heartiness of the spores of the *Clostridium* bacterium that can grow extremely well when plated under anaerobic conditions. This test, which must be ordered separately, finds its greatest application in the care of children with autism when the presence of *Clostridim* is indicated on the organic acids analysis, it grows on initial testing of the stool, or is otherwise suspected. It is commonly recognized that children with autism struggle with the overgrowth of this bacterium in their intestines and with the deleterious effects some species of *Clostridim* exert on their behavior. The fact that *Clostridium* constitute up to 30% of total colonic bacteria suggests that the actual amount of *Clostridium* species present may be underreported using conventional methodology, and that some of this species can be part of normal microbiota.

PARASITE TESTING

A major benefit of a stool examination is that it can detect the presence of parasites (including parasitic bacterial species) that are much more common in children with autism than is generally recognized. Recently, a test has become available that is reported to be able to identify intestinal organisms using their DNA. This gastrointestinal function profile is available through the Metametrix Clinical Laboratory.

SHORT CHAIN FATTY ACID TESTING

When the stool is subjected to chemical analysis, it provides additional useful information. This is the second part of the stool analysis test. It is not always requested because it increases the cost of the test. However, I recommend it be included initially as it can help with both diagnosis and management. The information provided includes stool pH (acid or alkaline) and the presence of blood or excess mucus. The test also reports the amount of beneficial short chain fatty acids (SCFA) that are necessary for the growth of good bacteria that protect the intestinal lining against the development of adult malignancy, especially colon cancer. In addition, the test also provides an assessment of the degree of intestinal inflammation, along with an indication of pancreatic function and fat digestion. This part of the stool analysis notes the presence of any undigested food, the amount of secretory

IgA (the intestinal border patrol molecule that is active against pathogens), and several other items.

LEAVE IT TO THE EXPERTS

The treatment of dysbiosis and the leaky gut is best left to experienced practitioners. The specifics of such management are beyond the scope of this discussion. Suffice it to say that each physician has his or her own approach that they have found successful. Very high doses of probiotics are currently in favor and some clinicians are using fewer prescription antibiotics and depending more on herbal agents, such as oil of oregano.

ANTIBODY TESTING

Blood testing can also be very helpful. One type of blood testing that can be requested is an antibody test used to detect food allergens. According to this theory, if the antibody test indicates a high amount of immunoglobulin G antibody (called IgG) in response to a particular food, it means the individual is allergic to that food. The body produces the IgG antibody in response to a food it considers harmful in the same manner that the body produces an antibody against a certain infectious disease, such as measles. This type of reaction is of the delayed type, meaning that it may take hours or days to manifest itself. When the number of foods evoking a high IgG antibody response skyrockets, this is a good indicator of the presence of a leaky gut.

IgG ANTIBODY TESTING

The blood tests that analyze the blood for foods which elevate the various food IgG antibodies are available through many testing laboratories, including the ones mentioned above. Note that eating a problem food frequently and close to the time of testing may cause a marked IgG response. Therefore, when a food only shows a minor IgG reactivity, it should not be taken lightly. This food could turn into a major offender if it is consumed frequently and in greater amounts.

TWO CAVEATS

Dr Liz Mumper of the Rimland Center stresses (and, I believe very correctly) that the primary treatment of food allergies is to restore integrity and health to the intestinal mucosa, in other words, repair the leaky gut wall. Simply eliminating foods that evoke a high IgG response is not the answer. In addition, some practitioners and scientists are not convinced of the usefulness of the IgG antibody test in assessing a person's food allergies.

IMMUNOGLOBULIN E ANTIBODY TESTING

A determination of the amount of immunoglobulin E antibody the body produces against various foods is available through Genova, DD, GPL, and other testing companies. This test reports foods which cause an immune reaction to develop seconds to minutes after they are eaten. Peanuts are an example. Such reactions can be life-threatening and, if their presence is suspected, it is advisable to consult with an allergist who has expertise in the diagnosis and treatment of such problems.

ALLERGY TESTING BY OTHERS

The classic and perhaps the simplest way to determine if one is allergic to a food is to eliminate that particular food and see if the allergic symptoms disappear. If this happens, the procedure is to reintroduce that food at a time when no other changes are being made in the regimen and see if the symptoms reappear. If they do recur when the food is again eaten, the allergy to that particular food is confirmed. This method usually can be used safely for evaluating foods which cause delayed symptoms. As noted above, evaluation of substances which cause an immediate, violent, even life-threatening reaction are best left to a medical specialist in the field of allergy and immunology.

Some IgG food reactions also manifest themselves shortly after the food is consumed. However, when an allergic reaction causes abrupt swelling in the form of hives, especially if breathing is affected, the condition becomes an emergency and an allergist should be consulted. Some cases may require a prompt visit to the Emergency Room or an Urgent Care Clinic.

SKIN TESTING

A popular means of diagnosing allergies with traditional doctors is called skin testing. An allergist applies a small amount of the test substance to or just under the skin. The specific methodology is beyond the scope of this book. The skin test can be used to check for many allergens, such as pollens, molds, animal dander, or foods.

ELECTROMERMAL TESTING

Electrodermal testing is another type of sensitivity testing for foods that in my experience has been quite reliable. In electrodermal testing, also called electro-acupuncture according to Voll (EAV), the changes in the electrical resistance of the skin are tested by a galvanometer connected to a computer as the body is exposed to signals from various foods. Electrodermal testing is non-invasive. The skin is not broken or penetrated. Some alternative medicine practices provide this test. It is critical that the operator be experienced with the use of this machine. Otherwise results will be inconsistent, confusing, and could result in a waste of precious resources by going down roads that are non-productive.

INHALANT TESTING

Sometimes I recommend considering a blood check for

o inhalants that enter the body through breathing. ..is test measures immunoglobulin E (IgE), which typically causes a more immediate adverse response. Such testing checks for IgE elevations against molds, dusts, trees, grasses, and even toxins, such as the mercury-containing preservative, thimerosal. Inhalants may be an even greater problem than foods for some individuals, and they also can be associated with dysbiosis and the leaky gut that follows. The existence of an inhalant allergy can allow an influx of additional allergenic substances into the bloodstream, such as partially digested foods, debris and poisons from disintegrating intestinal organisms, other chemicals in the gut, and even medications. One of my patients with autism, who was experiencing considerable allergic symptoms during the night, was found to have a dust mite allergy on the inhalant allergy test by GPL. Other foreign chemicals in the gut can include those new-to-nature additives used to adulterate food to make it more commercially attractive.

NO "NATURAL" FLAVORINGS

A food or any other substance that causes hives or a rash can also cause an equivalent reaction in the brain. When this circumstance exists within our central nervous system, the condition is sometimes called a "brain allergy." (37) This brain allergy occurs in some forms of migraine headache, and it is just as real an entity as an adverse reaction on the surface of the body, which we can more easily see. A brain allergy to a food additive is a common cause of hyperactivity in children. Therefore, it is not a good idea to feed an ASD child or one with ADHD any prepared or packaged food. If unable to follow this recommendation completely, at least become a label-reader, and especially read the fine print. Carefully research anything that appears in the ingredients, including abbreviations and umbrella terms such as "natural flavorings".

Many parents are surprised to learn that food producers consider some very unnatural chemicals to be "natural." Hyperreactivity of the body to those particular allergens requires measures to cool off or tone down the body's immune system. (This treatment will be addressed in Chapter Six.)

THE PULSE TEST

Twenty minutes or so after consuming an offending food, an increase in the pulse rate of four beats or more per minute may occur. I include this test here only as a matter of information. I do not recommend it because foods are better tested in an allergist's office which is equipped to deal with a severe allergic reaction that ingesting some foods, as peanuts or shellfish, could cause. And certainly, the testing of foods that are suspected --or known-- to cause hives or difficulty in breathing should never be attempted at home. Some years ago a physician who began using the pulse as a means of food sensitivity testing wrote a small book about his findings.(38)

OTHER INTOLERANCES

Certain foods can be harmful to individuals, even though they are not per se allergic to them. For example, some individuals cannot tolerate dairy foods that contain the sugar lactose because they lack the intestinal enzyme lactase needed to digest lactose. These lactose-intolerant individuals might have either inherited a condition or acquired one that causes them to lose their ability to make the lactase. In either case, to avoid unpleasant G-I symptoms such as gas and bloating, lactose-intolerant individuals must either avoid dairy products, purchase ones that are lactose-free, or use the enzyme lactase.

GET YOUR GOAT YET?

Research conducted on dairy goat milk composition at the University of California-Davis suggests the reason why some cow's milk-intolerant individuals can better tolerate goat's milk may lie in the fact that the type of lactalbumin present in goat's milk elicits less of an allergic response compared with that in cow's milk. The researchers note that such allergies are serious problems especially for young children.*

A WORD TO THE WISE

Avoiding dairy products altogether might make one deficient in the mineral calcium that has many important functions in the body. This situation would require an adequate supply of calcium from other food choices or by taking calcium in supplement form. Because milk is also rich in beneficial phosphorous, supplying phosphorous in some other form is also necessary.

OXALATES --SOMETHING TO BE DEALT WITH

Of the many aspects of autism, oxalates are perhaps the most misunderstood. And yet, these unwelcome natural chemicals may play a key role in ASDs and in many other conditions such as fibromyalgia, intersititial cystitis, depression, arthritis, and gut problems --to name a few. For example, the presence of too many oxalates in the G-I tract from eating a regular diet, or following a specific carbohydrate diet from which high-oxalate foods have not been removed, may kill the beneficial organisms despite administration of huge probiotic doses. Oxalates can also interfere with the roles of magnesium, zinc, iron, and other body ions. And if sulfur metabolism is awry (another common problem in autism), the transporting of oxlates in the kidney, intestine, and even the brain may be affected, and pathways that make oxalates in the body may be accelerated.

HOW DID WE MISS THIS?

First, many scientists incorrectly believe oxalates only cause problems in the kidneys, such as stones. So that's where most

*http://www.drinc.ucdavis.edu/**goat**1.htm

of the research has been conducted. Also, measuring oxalates in the urine (the most common way in which they are determined) will not reveal a high blood oxalate that may be present irrespective of the urinary oxalate value. This hyperoxalemia, as it is called, may be an indication that these natural toxins are being formed within the body. Oxalate may accumulate due to deficiencies of vitamin B-6 (pyridoxine) or vitamin B-1 (thiamine), or from a genetic biochemical pathway abnormality. In one important study, the blood oxalate level of children with autism was threefold higher that that of unaffected children.(39)

GOOD GUYS AND BAD GUYS

All human beings lack the enzyme that allows them to metabolize oxalates. Oxalates are found in nuts, spinach, chocolate --among other foods-- and in some herbs and medications. Therefore, it is incorrect to view oxalates as a problem for only some people. They may cause damage in the bodies (including the brains) of everyone who lacks normal intestinal flora, including *Oxalobacer formigines*. These intestinal bacteria have the capacity to digest oxalates, thereby changing them into a less irritating and harmful form. As of this writing, supplementing this organism is still in research stages. However, high dose *Lactobacillus acidophilus* and high dose mixed *Lactobacillus* probiotic formulations that can reduce oxalate levels are commercially available.

Be forewarned: antibiotics kill beneficial intestinal bacteria and exact their price. The cost? Dysbiosis can develop and along with it a leaky gut. Oxalates further complicate matters.

WHAT HELPS

We humans are therefore dependent on the right intestinal flora to digest oxalates, thus preventing their absorption into the body where they can disturb organ function, including brain function. Oxalates preferentially accumulate in organs that have already been damaged. In predisposed individuals --the number of whom we may greatly underestimate-- management consists of avoiding high-oxalate foods. Also, if the individual is in oxidative stress, in other words, when a great deal of tissue damage is occurring due to excessive free radical activity, high doses of vitamin C should be avoided because vitamin C can form oxalates. Another effective approach is to ingest a moderate amount of calcium citrate before every meal. Calcium will tie up the oxalates in the G-I tract and prevent their absorption. In addition, calcium promotes closure of the between-the-cells gap of a leaky gut.

GOOD NEWS

Treating a leaky gut is therefore paramount. Otherwise oxalates will be absorbed into the body from the stomach and through the small bowel's leaky wall before the appropriate intestinal bacteria residing downstream in the colon have an opportunity to digest them. Not only will treating a leaky gut prevent harmful oxalates from being absorbed, they will also remain in the gut until they reach the colon where they can be properly degraded. Should allergy testing disclose a large number of problem foods, you may assume oxalates are being absorbed as well. Conversely, experience has shown that effective management of the oxalate problem has resulted in a huge decrease in the number of problem foods on repeat food sensitivity testing. Improvements in sociability and language in children with autism have also been reported.

My source for this information was oxalate specialist Susan Costen Owens of the Autism Oxalate Project. She also has kindly provided the literature reference cited above (39) and two internet links describing this topic in greater detail. (40,41) Your review of this informative material will be time well-spent.

SALICYLATES

Salicylates are another group of chemicals to which some people are sensitive and should avoid. Aspirin, apples, wine, and many other foods contain these salicylates. Practitioners familiar with treating allergies can determine whether or not an individual is sensitive to salicylates.

SULFITES

Finally, some people are intolerant of sulfites, commonly found in dried fruit, wine, and other foods. Sulfites are also present in some mists applied over salad bars to maintain freshness. The internet provides lists of foods according to their oxalate, salicylate, and sulfite content.

HOW TO FIX EVERTHING

Dear reader, you might at this point ask in bewilderment, "Then what is left to eat?" Please be patient and keep any discouragement at bay. There is a way out of all this, and its name is "Heal the Gut!" Another equally important solution also exists. It involves the immune system and the liver. If operating properly, the liver will process and inactivate foreign materials entering the body. However, if the liver is overburdened with toxins and "new-to-nature molecules" its function will falter. The task of dealing with the onslaught of all these foreign antigens entering through the G-I tract will then be thrust upon the immune system. (What this important body system is and does will be covered in a later chapter). For now it's sufficient to say the immune system may react to this increased work load by going into in a state of alarm. The consequence is hyperreactivity distributed over the whole body. And systemic symptoms, such as allergies and others described above that we ascribe to the presence of a leaky gut, will start popping up. Much more of the liver's role in all this will be covered later. Here we simply note that if the liver is functioning efficiently as a filter, its bloodstream-cleansing effect will decrease the strain on the immune system. In addition, because the liver is a storehouse of vitamins and healing substances, a healthy liver is able to provide the nutrients needed to heal the G-I tract and repair the leaky gut so that fewer foreign molecules gain admission to the body. As a consequence of the liver's activity, the body can down-regulate its sensitivity to foreign proteins, so food allergies can begin to fade away. My hope is that by persistence you will learn much about this topic and, in the end, be rewarded with a workable plan for your child.

CASEIN AND GLUTEN SENSITIVITY

Gluten is a protein found in grains, such as wheat, rye, and barley. Casein is a protein found in milk and related milk products, such as cheese and sometimes yogurt. All people are unable to properly digest gluten and/or casein. They suffer unpleasant reactions of various sorts when consuming foods containing these proteins. The solution is a diet free from the gluten or casein or both. Avoiding gluten and/or casein has greatly benefited many individuals who are sensitive to one or both of those proteins. Unfortunately, this measure is not as easy as it sounds. Many processed foods contain gluten and/or casein. Because wheat has been thought of from time immemorial as being the staff of life, it finds its way into many of the foods people eat daily. And casein is used as a filler in hot dogs and many other sausage meats.

FIRST TO TRY

As previously discussed, a number of doctors and researchers have found that poor digestion significantly contributes to autism and ADHD. Since gluten and casein sensitivity are common causes of poor digestion in the general population, it's reasonable that these sensitivities be considered in managing persons with autism and ADHD. Avoidance of at least gluten is a common intervention, and it certainly has reaped many rewards. This matter is not without controversy, but I believe in its validity.

USUALLY WORKS

Many traditional practitioners cite references in medical literature that claim there is no benefit to eliminating casein and gluten from the diets of children with autism. They argue that gluten-free (G/F) and casein-free (C/F) diets are expensive and worthless. On the other hand, as noted by Dr. Sidney Baker, there have been published success stories of treating both schizophrenia and autism with gluten-free diets dating back as far as fifty years. (42) In addition, many other practitioners experience remarkable success in treating autism by removing gluten and casein. Because of this successful track record, complementary practitioners often recommend a G/F-C/F diet as their first intervention. As noted, these diets, often, but not always, have a beneficial effect on the health of children with autism and ADHD.

GUT-BRAIN CONNECTION

The old observation that schizophrenia, as well as autism, improve when gluten is removed from the diet hints at the brain-gut connection. (42) This intriguing connection was researched and reported on by Dr. Michael Gershon in his landmark book on this subject entitled *The Second Brain*. (43) The understanding of the gut-brain connection has been further advanced through work in Dr. Martha G. Welch's laboratory at Columbia College of Physicians and Surgeons in New York. I am excited to share the results of her key discovery with you at the end of this chapter.

THE PEPTIDE STORY

Why is gluten, and sometimes casein, harmful to some individuals? Gluten and casein molecules resemble long chains folded upon themselves. Uniquely, they contain unusually large amounts of the amino acid proline. Our own protein-digesting enzymes, called proteases, disassemble these molecular chains into fragments, called peptides, each containing eight amino acids. But it's up to another enzyme group called peptidases to complete the breakdown process to individual amino acids which then can be absorbed into the body and used as building blocks for the structural proteins that make up our tissues and enzymes.(42)

DPP4 is the name given to the peptidase charged with this final disassembly process. It is well suited for this task because it has the capacity to cleave the many interconnecting bonds created by the large amount of proline present.

However, DPP4 activity can suffer from environmental toxicity. This was discovered some years ago in a study that investigated DPP4 activity in human placenta. The investigators found that the enzymatic activity of DPP4 was greatly diminished by the presence of mercury (mercuric chloride), organophosphates (pesticide sprays), zinc, cadmium chlorides, and lead acetate. (47) This means a person may be unable to digest gluten and casein because the toxins present in their bodies inactivated the enzyme that would normally assist in this task.

You don't need to have metal toxicity to have sensitivity to gluten or casein. Nobody breaks down gluten or casein efficiently, but this type of food intolerance can certainly coexist with celiac disease and complicate the management of both disorders.

TROUBLEMAKERS

The undigested peptides from gluten and casein cause mischief in the body in two ways. First of all they bear a similarity with at least some human tissue, for example, intestinal lining cells. The result is that any immune response against these protein fragments can attack some of our body tissues as well.(42)

Secondly, instead of remaining in the intestine, some of the undigested peptides enter the bloodstream. Here, because of their molecular and functional resemblance to opium or morphine, they behave like narcotics and "dock" with opioid receptors in the brain, thereby addicting an individual under these circumstances to the very foods that are bad for them. This whole problem escalates in the presence of a leaky gut. (42)

These persons then crave foods, such as pizza, that contains both gluten in the crust and casein in the cheese topping. Does this addiction sound familiar? This is especially true for predisposed individuals, such as those with autism or ADHD.

Use of the word "addiction" is not an overstatement. Dramatic withdrawl symptoms can occur in individuals, including children, when they come off gluten. The malaise and irritability strongly resemble a mild version of what occurs in heroin withdrawl. (42) A few of my patients have experienced this reaction. Fortunately, it lasted only a few hours.

Adulterants in packaged pizza, including food dyes, preservatives, artificial flavorings, flavor enhancers, and other chemicals can also do a significant amount of damage to vulnerable, developing brains.

CELIAC DISEASE

Celiac disease is caused by an inherited mix of genes that contribute to a heightened immune sensitivity to gluten that results in damaging the intestinal lining cells. Gliadin, casein (from diary products), and a host of other proteins may not be tolerated because their molecular configuration resembles gluten. Thus, the body reacts to them as it would to gluten. The more gluten-intolerant an individual, the longer the list of problem foods. For more on this situation, called molecular mimicry, refer to Dr. Thomas O'Bryan's research that is well-described on his educational C.D.(44)

Once again, I recommend Dr. Fasano's article on celiac disease published in *Scientific American* magazine. (35) This is a "must read" for anyone interested in G-I disorders and the systemic impact these disorders can have. According to a study conducted by Barcia and colleagues, ASD children were found to have a three-fold higher prevalence of celiac disease than the general pediatric population. For this reason, the investigators suggested that all ASD children should be screened for celiac disease by blood testing, whether or not GI symptoms are present. (45)

NOT CELIAC BUT STILL NOT WELL

I wish this discussion could end here but first I want to note that sensitivity to gluten that is not due to celiac disease does indeed exist and as yet isn't very well understood. It is more common than celiac disease and lies midway in the sensitivity spectrum between an allergic reaction to wheat mediated by IgE antibodies (which cause immediate allergic symptoms, such as hives and congestion) at one extreme and celiac disease at the other.

Non-celiac gluten sensitivity doesn't exhibit the classic damage to intestinal lining cells that is seen in celiac patients, nor does it include, per se, a leaky gut. It appears to involve a more primitive immune response than is present in celiac patients, and resembling the mechanism described above in the paragraph subtitled TROUBLEMAKERS. Like celiac disease, it can be associated with both intestinal symptoms (bloating, diarrhea, abdominal pain, and diarrhea) and extraintestinal symptoms (migraine, fatigue, and ADHD). However, the systemic damage in celiac disease, such as osteoporosis, short stature, and brain degeneration can be more permanent.

FASTING FROM HARMFUL FOODS

If the cells lining the inside of the intestine (mucosal cells) become damaged by dysbiosis (from yeast, parasitic, or bacterial overgrowth) or an immune reaction to gluten or related proteins, they lose their ability to perform the last step of digestion by enzymes called disaccharidases. These enzymes break down two sugar molecules hooked together (called disaccharides) and also many starches (called poly-saccharides). In this event, the G-I tract sustains further damage and loss of function. For recovery to occur other foods, besides those containing gluten and casein must be removed from the diet. These include lactose (milk sugar), sucrose (table sugar), maltose sugars, corn, millet, oats, all rice, all types of potatoes, soybeans (and food containing soy), garbanzo beans, wheat germ, and most substitute flours. (29)

SPECIAL FOOD REGIMEN

A word of encouragement is appropriate here. Disaccharides and starches may need to be omitted for a time, but Elaine Gotschall in her book lists food choices and provides a large number of recipes based on these food choices. It would certainly be worth trying this regimen with your child because it might finally subdue a stubborn yeasty overgrowth and restore intestinal health. (29) Finally, this approach allows some foods that are taboo in the G/F C/F diet, such as certain cheeses. AND these restrictions do not last forever.

CEREBRAL FOLATE DEFICIENCY

An additional reason for omitting cow's milk from the diet is the finding that in some children its removal decreases the formation of antibodies against the "dock" or receptor, where folic acid attaches in the brain. Folic acid, the prime source of which is green leafy vegetables, is part of an essential biochemical process called methylation. The brain disorder stemming from lack of folic acid is called "cerebral folate deficiency" (CFD). Supplementing folic acid to children with this disorder resulted in improvements in some of the children in areas of muscular coordination, seizure frequency, communication, and repetitious movements (called stereotypy). However, in doses greater than 200-300mcg folic acid may actually exhibit anti-folate effects* Administration of the related substance, folinic acid, can enter the folate cycle and improve motor skills in children with CFD (48) But folinic acid is not an active folate. The best folate supplement is methylfolate. Some interesting information appears on a 5/11/12 entry on the website noted below* Laboratory testing for genes that interfere with formation of methylfolate are widely available and frequently are covered by standard insurance plans. This information is so important that this testing is listed first on the newborn testing suggestions in Appendix D.

MORE RESOURCES

An treatment outline for these intestinal problems

* mthfr.net/mthfr-testing-mthfr-testkit/2012/01/25/

has been discussed in this chapter. This excellent care plan is available online under the title *A More Complete Approach to G-I Suppot, the "4-R Program"*. The program has four parts. Phase 1 includes removal of offending substances, such as the foods that are not tolerated from the diet. Phase 2 stresses replacement of digestive enzymes and gastric acid when necessary. Phase 3 interventions are to re-inoculate the bowel with pre- and probiotics. (Prebiotics are special kinds of dietary fiber on which the probiotic organisms grow). And in Phase 4, proper nutritional support is provided in order to regenerate the G-I mucosa. This protocol is best implemented under the guidance of a health care provider who understands and appreciates the critical role that G-I health plays in general health and well being. (49)

PROBLEM SOLVED

The consequences of proper dietary treatment can be excellent. Abdominal pain, bloating, cramping, diarrhea, and constipation can be relieved and the "leaky gut" greatly improved. In addition, the resulting restoration of the digestive process causes the number of foods that are not tolerated to characteristically plummet. Of course, it may be necessary to temporarily avoid the foods that caused the problem to begin with, such as carbohydrates, foods containing gluten and casein, and sometimes foods containing corn and soy.

Not only do the intestines heal, but with appropriate attention, other organs of digestion heal as well. For example, the liver, stomach, and pancreas will provide a better quality and quantity of digestive juices. Furthermore, if toxic metals and chemicals were inactivating DPP4, then the removal of these toxins and their elimination from the body should result in some return of DPP4 function and allow gradual reintroduction of some gluten- and casein-containing foods. The elimination of toxic metals and chemicals will be addressed in Chapters Four and Six.

INTESTINAL AND BRAIN INFLAMMATION ASSOCIATION

I close this chapter by relating a vital discovery alluded to above that was made by Dr. Welch and her colleagues. When this research group induced inflammatory bowel disease (in humans it would be called Crohn's disease) in experimental animals, they noted that as the intestine inflamed, so did the brain. Even more importantly, as the intestinal inflammation decreased with treatment, so did brain inflammation. The paper notes that both the intestine and the brain are derived from the same embryonic tissue and that parts of both organs have receptors for the hormones secretin and oxytocin. Therefore, this association of inflammation in both the brain and the gut and its disappearance with treatment may be explained by the common tissue origin of these organs. (50)

FIX THE BELLY AND HEAL THE BRAIN

These findings have important implications for the management of autism because intestinal disease is so very common in ASD, and autism is also very much a disorder of the brain. The prospect of being able to control inflammation in brain cells by effectively managing the causes of intestinal inflammation and the associated gut infection provides reasonable hope that brain function will improve as inflammation in that organ lessens. Many reports document inflamed intestines in ASD. Other reports cite inflammation in the brain of persons with autism. Welch's research with live animals sheds light on the causation and mechanism of the link between inflammation in these two organs, as well as presenting plausible principles of treatment.

BENEFIT OF MATERNAL NURTURING

Many students of this subject believe that intestinal inflammation appears first. It is also possible that the inflammation in the brain cells is the initial event, and then the intestinal cells became inflamed. Welch's findings may provide an explanation for this. She is not only a scientist, but a psychiatrist. She has been investigating the importance of maternal nurturing early in life. She has especially researched the benefits of ample maternal nurturing in the NICU setting. The finding that this nurturing decreases inflammation in the newborn brain would add credence to the premise that brain inflammation occurred first, followed by intestinal inflammation responding to messenger molecules originating in the brain and reaching the intestine through the bloodstream. Thus, the increase in healing hormones, oxytocin and secretin, in response to breastfeeding and lovingly holding the baby, would simultaneously decrease inflammation in the brain and the gut. (50) (See the discussion of the birthing process discussed earlier in this chapter.)

INCREASING OXYTOCIN --THE BOTTOM LINE

Managing intestinal problems in some children with autism using only a GI- based approach without addressing what is occurring in a child's brain might not result in healing either organ or in a general improvement in the autistic condition. This being the case, what is the solution to treating older children, or even adults? What can be done to help nurture them, even if maternal nurturing --by far the optimal form of nurturing-- isn't possible? There is another approach that stimulates the same hormones that maternal nurturing does. This measure might help individuals with autism of all ages. This concept is based on research conducted on how primitive man was able to domesticate animals. This research reveals a significant increase in the amount of oxytocin in both the human and the animal involved in the domestication process. (51)

CONTINUING OXYTOCIN RELEASE

As noted above, both the intestinal tract and the brain have receptors for oxytocin and secretin. Clinical studies have demonstrated that the administration of secretin to some children with autism, either intravenously or by nasal spray, can be associated with symptomatic improvement. In my limited experience, this is also true for oxytocin when it is administered as a nasal spray. Is it possible that a close, loving and ongoing association with animals could ameliorate autism by means of continuous oxytocin release? I will discuss this fascinating possibility in Chapter Five of this book entitled *"Help From The Barn"*.

Chapter Four

Dark Skies and Dirty Water

The Problem

IT'S ALL STACKING UP

The last chapter identified intestinal dysbiosis as an enemy within the body that poisons it. This chapter will discuss the modern environment in which we live as another source of poison. In actuality, our modern environment is an external enemy that is of equal or even greater importance than the enemy within. And the strength of this environmental enemy is growing more menacing each day.

IS AUTISM ENVIRONMENTAL?

If that question could be answered with a definitive "yes", then the explanation currently espoused by many, including our government, that the meteoric rise in the incidence of autism is mostly ascribable to better diagnostic methods, would be once and for all be disproven. In this chapter, and in those that follow, golden threads of truth linking autism to an unsafe environment will surface. Supporting evidence from different sources will intertwine and, hopefully by the end of this book, we will have in hand a palpable fabric of reality. Not only is the answer "Yes, the cause of autism is largely, but not completely, environmental." However, the solution to this horrific problem now lies on our doorstep. We must be open to it.

JUST A LITTLE BIT WILL DO

Addressing environmental dangers in a book about autism is essential because the metabolic machinery (located largely in the liver) that processes and excretes toxins is compromised in autism. (2,8) This means that a person with this affliction responds to a small amount of environmental poison as if it were a very large amount. In this chapter we will justify the need to identify the modern environment as an enemy for persons with autism and ADHD and, likely, for all of us as well. Let us try to understand the magnitude of environmental dangers by presenting some related realities.

SHOCKING NEWS

To begin with, an ongoing study in a large U.S. city discovered that one third of all tested children were developmentally delayed. This study also found that hundreds (yes, hundreds!) of polluting chemicals were found in umbilical cord blood of American newborns of every social strata, even though more than two thirds of these chemicals had been banned from the market for years. This certainly makes one wonder where these poisons had been hiding and accumulating in the interim.(52-54)

MORE SHOCKING NEWS

Next, consider the magnitude of this problem in the following example. An ingredient in the largest selling herbicide in the

U.S that was touted as being harmless has now been shown to kill human cells.(55,56). Worse, this herbicidal ingredient is especially poisonous to embryonic cells at doses well below the levels that are commonly found in food.(57) Cells from an organism at the earliest stages of its development, well before birth, are called embryonic cells. Later in this chapter, this herbicide will be discussed in more detail, and with good reason: about 100 million pounds of this weed killer are applied each year in the United States alone.(58)

IS ANYONE IN CONTROL?

A national report issued over 70 years ago stated that the amount of organic matter in some soils had already dropped too low to support efficient farming.(59) In truth, the chemicalized agriculture that mushroomed after World War II has now contaminated our farm soil that already had been nutrient-depleted for decades. Consequences of such contaminations include the finding that four and five year old children who resided in a heavily pesticided valley lost both their gross and fine hand-eye coordination and did not posses an adequate memory of recent events. When these unfortunate children were asked to draw the figure of a person, they could only produce a series of disconnected lines. Drawings by counterpart children from surrounding hills that were not sprayed were normal.(52)

The above findings are very troubling and prompt one to wonder whether the problems with our environment and our farmland can be quickly solved, especially since experience reveals that these problems are very difficult to remediate. And so is the damage they do. Dr. Philip Landrigan, who is Dean for Global Health at the Mount Sinai School of Medicine in New York, reported that neurodevelopmental disabilities are for the most part permanent and irreversible. Treatment of these environmentally caused neurobehavioral disorders is very difficult. In most cases, lifelong treatment is required. The cost of these disorders to the United States is conservatively estimated to be 52.6 billion dollars each year. Landrigan stated that a current ban on the chemicals causing these disabilities is costly, inefficient, and a late strategy to prevent damage to the human brain. He recommends pre-market testing of these chemicals before they are released into the environment, especially because infant's and children's brains are exquisitely sensitive to toxic substances. Exposure early in life may predispose to the development of Alzheimer's and Parkinson's disease in adulthood.(60)

Unfortunately, none of these findings are imaginary. This is the world we live in and the "dark skies and dirty water" are becoming darker and dirtier --and, I fear, ever more damaging-- every day.

POLLUTION VS AUTISM

Not long ago, Martha Herbert, PhD, MD from Harvard Medical School's Massachusetts General Hospital made a presentation concerning the relationship between the development of autism and adverse environmental conditions. Dr. Herbert focused on our ecosystem (the relationship between organisms and their environment) and how its deterioration impacts autism. She explained that the U.S. production of chemicals and plastics increases each year. She displayed a graph that depicted the climbing rates of chemicals and production of plastics during the 1990's and compared it to a very similar looking graph showing the climbing rates of autism during the same period.(52)

IT'S EVERYWHERE

Next, Herbert discussed some studies that showed that heavy metals, such as lead, cadmium, and mercury can be detected in newborn meconium or in umbilical cord blood. She noted that these studies also indicated the presence of many pesticides and even cancer-causing agents, such as polycyclic aromatic hydrocarbons, in umbilical cord blood. These studies made it clear that fetal exposure to environmental toxins is not only present but also prevalent. In fact, at a recent environmental toxicity meeting, Herbert stated that our newborns are already entoxified with metals, industrial chemicals, and pesticides, 287 of them, at birth. (53) Worse still, she noted that nearly 200 of these substances have been banned from the market for years. (54)

EVEN BENEATH OUR FEET

Where have these dangerous substances been all this time? What situation allows their unrecognized persistence and still permits them to find their way into the blood stream of unborn babies while they are still in their mother's womb? The answer partly appears to be that, as far as pesticides are concerned, they have been buried in our cropland and have gained entrance into our bodies through the food chain. These agricultural chemicals also have been accumulating in human liver and fatty tissue and in the organs of animals as well.(61) In Chapter Six I will present evidence that supports such storage. And later in this chapter, I will provide another explanation of how dangerous substances have been deposited into our farming soil.

WHAT GOOD ARE LAWS IF THEY AREN'T FOLLOWED?

A particularly scary and seemingly irresponsible part of all this is how infrequently the Environmental Protection Agency (EPA) or the manufacturers themselves conduct toxicity testing on these chemicals. Of the 2,863 chemicals produced in excess of one million pounds annually, Herbert showed that only 12 of them, a meager 0.4 %, have been tested for neurodevelopmental toxicity according to EPA guidelines. Autism is an example of a human neurodevelopmental disorder. For a little over 20% of these chemicals, some data exists on developmental toxicity, but there is no data at all on the developmental toxicity in over 78% of the chemicals being produced by the ton daily.(52) Developmental toxicity is a term to describe any factor that interferes with how an embryo matures into its adult form. In this setting, it refers to experiments conducted on animals or other living creatures in the laboratory. However in real life situations, these chemicals are collecting in our environment and causing dark skies and dirty water, accumulating in animal and human tissues, and they are also building up in our children at a time when they are being formed in the womb! (61)

WHAT MORE PROOF DO WE NEED?

Developmental abnormalities occur early when the child is still in the womb. This is especially relevant in view of the exquisite vulnerability of the developing human brain to toxic chemicals in the environment. (60) The causal link between environmental contamination and the rising rates of autism can be inferred by comparing two maps that Herbert presented. These maps depicted the incidence of autism in all the school districts in Texas obtained from Department of Education records in conjunction with maps depicting the quantity of chemicals produced in Texas, by county.(52) This latter information was obtained from the Toxic Release Inventory (TRI). Federal law requires the EPA and the individual states to collect data annually on the releases and transfers of certain toxic chemicals from industrial facilities, including mines, and make this data available to the public through the TRI.(62)

If one compares the reported autism rates from 1990-1993 with those reported in 1998-2000, one notices a startling increase in autism in the latter years. School districts with low autism rates were represented in white on the map, those with intermediate autism rates in gray, and those with high rates in black. Whereas most of the districts were portrayed in white or gray in 1990-1993, by the time of the second report, half of the state had turned black. This means that about half the school districts in Texas reported high rates of autism.(52) That study is now 11 years old. And the incidence of autism has continued to rise sharply since then. Our government reports that in the United States, as of 2008, one in every 54 eight year old boys --or 1 in 110 eight year old children-- suffers from autism. This document, which was released in 2012, also noted that, in the 2003-4 school year, 1% of all British children, aged 5-9, were similarly affected. (63)

When one compares the maps of autism by school district with the amount of chemicals produced in those counties from the TRI reports, one can clearly see that that the areas of high autism rates are in the same areas where there is the most environmental chemical release and transfer. Although the correlation between these two statistics doesn't definitively prove causation, it certainly provides a strong incentive to determine the reasons for this high correlation.(52)

HOW MANY OF THE 2,863?

On the positive side, in what many consider to be a long-overdue measure, Herbert quoted a source stating that the EPA would soon release a list of the toxins that are likely to play a role in autism and other neurological disorders. The preliminary draft of this list of toxins includes methylmercury, aluminum, arsenic, bisphenol A, cadmium, DEET, lead, PCB's, and phthalates. Sadly --but not unexpectedly-- after one year, six congressional hearings, and 10 "stakeholder sessions", the proposed legislation was dead. This is a cogent testament to the combined clout of the $674 billion chemical industry. (64) At least some of the poisons listed above are included in the Texas TRI. In support of Herbert's postulate that the presence of these toxins is causing autism, she quoted research conducted at the University of Texas Health Science Center and the San Antonio Department of Family and Community Medicine. This research revealed that, on the average, for every 1,000 pounds of environmentally released mercury, there was a 61% increase in the rate of autism in Texas. Mercury is only one of many contaminants that are polluting the state of Texas.(52)

SOMEONE BETTER DO SOMETHING FAST

The final part of Herbert's presentation reported an assessment of our ecosystem that was sponsored in the year 2000 by the United Nations. The news was grim. Scientists reported that the damage to the ecosystem was so severe that they could no longer be confident that the earth would be able to support human life for more than two generations.(author's note: about 66 years). A recent update of our ecosystem, also commissioned by the U.N., states "The conclusion of the UN Millennium Ecosystem Assessment are clear: human activity is fundamentally and extensively changing the world around us, leading to extinction on a massive scale. The extent of human loss should not be underestimated. It points to a potential sixth great extinction on par with historic global extinctions caused by asteroid impacts."(65)

IS HUMANITY IN DANGER OF EXTINCTION?

How could such an obliteration of human life occur in a little over 50 years? A well-documented worldwide loss of fertility that is already being experienced in animals and humans alike may be the explanation.(66) Fifty years ago, the total fertility rate in the United States was 3.8 children per woman. Now, excluding immigrants, it is 1.9 children per woman, a figure that is below replacement rate.(67) Because many factors besides environmental toxicity appear to be influencing the decrease in the fertility rate, using the decrease in the sperm count may be a more useful measure of human reproductive failure.(66)

Environmental contamination with plastics and pesticides that either have estrogenic activity or in some other fashion interfere with female hormone function, along with the widespread increase in human obesity, are likely to be major reasons why the sperm count in Western industrialized countries has dropped more than 50% in the past 50 years. In other words, a male living in today's Western world requires the presence of both testicles to produce the same number of sperm that a male five decades ago could produce with only one testicle. Ironically, younger men have the poorest quality semen. A study in the 1990's found a decline in the human sperm count of about 2% yearly. If the decline continues at this rate, in just a few decades it will have dropped below 20 million sperms per ml. An individual with a sperm count of less than 20 million is considered to be infertile. Both male infertility and autism are linked to contamination of our environment. Thus it could be said that our failure to effectively and expeditiously address the environmental causes of autism will result in a large scale loss of the human species due to another manifestation of this contamination: widespread male infertility.(66)

PROFIT OVER HUMAN LIFE

Regarding the loss of human fertility, chemicals of concern are PCB's (used in electronics), vehicle exhaust fumes, pthalates leaching from plastics and used in dental fillings, man-made estrogen drugs, and pesticides such as DDE (made inside the body after exposure to DDT), atrazine, dieldrin, lindane, pentachlorophenol, and toxaphene. The most toxic man-made chemicals are dioxins. These are unwanted by-products of certain industrial processes, and we will encounter them again later in this book. DDT has been banned in the United States from the early 1970's, but it is still present in the body fat of all of us and new factories are still being built in India to produce DDT.(66) In a complete --and I submit morally wrong-- disregard of all of the foregoing, companies are continuing to produce chemicals in record amounts even though these chemicals, such as pesticides, plastics, and toxic metals are known to be human poisons. Consider how three northern New Jersey counties are contaminated with a highly poisonous form of chromium by irresponsible industrial practices beginning nearly a century ago. This continues to occur in the face of clear evidence that this metal is harmful to people exposed to it. See Appendix B for a current report on this environmental disaster and its possible association with autism.

WORLD-WIDE PROBLEM

Every day, more of these poisons are added to our environment. They are severely and, we are told, irreparably damaging our ecosystem. Our precious children are subjected to these poisons while they are still in the womb at a time when they are most vulnerable to being damaged. Is what we call autism a prime manifestation of that damage? The correlation between toxic environments and high autism rates is not limited to the United States. A South Korean study revealed that phthalates --chemicals widely used as softeners in plastics-- may reduce the IQ of grade school age boys and may alter brain development. (68) In that country now 1 in 38 children develop autism.(69) The daughter of a friend of mine who teaches English in South Korea notes that the pollution problem there may be worsened by airborne industrial waste contaminants from China.

In determining the incidence of autism in Korea, care was taken to screen every child, aged 7-12, in Ilsan, a community of nearly one half million persons. This is in contrast to the detection methods used by most research groups in the U.S. that measure autism prevalence based on records of existing cases from health care and special education agencies. To illustrate how these two methods of data collection differ, imagine an automobile manufacturer reporting the extent of a defect in a certain model based on each one of these models being examined during a massive recall, versus reporting the commonness of the problem based only on the number of defective cars that failed in service due to the defect. Thus, reporting the prevalence of autism based on the number of diagnosed cases may result in an erroneous underestimation of its true incidence. Thus many more children may be affected with autism than current reports indicate.

The world was shocked in 1989 when TV images taken in Copsa Mica, Romania showed black toxic soot from chimneys of a rubber-dye factory falling onto houses, fields, grazing sheep, and townspeople.(70) Did this toxin affect Romania's people? Dr. Martha Welch cites a study that reported a high incidence of developmental disorders --including autism-- in Romanian orphans from the 1980's and 1990's.(71) One in three children in that group were affected! There may be an additional intriguing reason why these orphans developed autism. This hypothesis was alluded to at the end of the last chapter and will be addressed again in Chapter Six.

WHAT ARE YOU HAVING FOR DINNER TONIGHT?

In light of all this information, one might wonder about our food supply. That at least should be safe, right? Unfortunately, it is far from safe. For example, Diane Olson Rutter reported that many toxins are present in the fertilizers used to produce our food. She wrote: "A sickening flow of heavy metals, nerve gas residue, dioxin, PCBs, pesticides, industrial solvents, petroleum oils and radioactive plutonium, americium, radium and strontium-90 makes its way from the Lowry Landfill Superfund site southeast of Denver, down 17 miles of pipe, and into the Denver Metro sewage treatment plant. There it joins the city's domestic and industrial waste and comes out the other end as sludge. Almost unbelievably, this sludge is then used to fertilize wheat." Later in the article she notes that this "fertilizer" is also used on grain crops used to make "specialty baked goods" by bakeries across the country.(72)

DILUTION IS NOT THE SOLUTION

Rutter also reported that the majority of the over 100 nations at the Basel Convention voted to prevent the United States from exporting its hazardous waste to poorer countries under the guise of fertilizer. But here at home the Resource Conservation and Recovery Act (RCRA) allows the addition of industrial and mining waste to fertilizer. This industrial waste includes ingredients such as plutonium, arsenic, mercury, cadmium, lead, PCBs, and dioxin that are taken from tailings, sumps, holding ponds, furnaces, and even from pollution control devices. The rationale used to justify the inclusion of this hazardous waste in fertilizer is that it also contains elements such as minerals that are beneficial to plant growth.(72)

THE PROBLEM IS REAL!

I was initially made aware of how this catastrophe plays out by another physician and friend who attended a soil seminar presented by a Minnesota firm, International Ag Labs, Inc. in 2003 in Kansas City. This doctor owns some acreage and wanted to learn effective means of restoring health to his farm soil. During this three day seminar, one of the speakers reported on methods to restore “dying” fields. The speaker described the typical scenario when a farmer begins to notice areas of his fields where crops and even other growth ceases. The following year more areas display the same signs. When the problem becomes so pervasive that it becomes apparent to the farmer that the crop yield will not even cover the input costs, he contacts this consulting firm. A soil analysis to determine the presence of any toxic metal or chemical that has built up in the soil in a quantity sufficient to prevent growth is obtained first. Then, the firm recommends a recovery program usually consisting of natural soil amendments or other biologic interventions that have been found to be effective to restore fertility in the situation under consideration. The speaker added that sometimes the soil is so laden with toxins as to be unremediable, or that the treatment cost could not be justified. He explained that the success of the soil revitalization program depends on what contaminants had been placed on the soil in past decades by repeated dressings of artificial fertilizer.(73)

The contaminants he referred to were the fillers added to the solid or liquid fertilizers. The fillers used are usually common to the area, based on the proximity of chemical plants or industrial operations that sell, give, or pay the fertilizer company to dispose of the hazardous waste products by spreading it on the farm land by way of fertilizer fillers. All these operations are supposedly in accord with the RCRA mentioned above. Sewage sludge that may have a similar list of ingredients --and in addition contain dangerous levels of disease-producing microorganisms-- can also be legally sold to farmers, home gardeners, or spread on public lands such as golf courses, parks, and playgrounds. (72)

It seems that industry, instead of properly disposing of its hazardous waste, has immorally and irresponsibly chosen to make money by selling it. This is done despite the fact that investigators of this activity have cited a growing number of cases across the country of injury, harm, and even death from exposure to sludge, primarily from the pathogen (infectious) content.(72)

HOW MUCH PROOF DO WE NEED?

While the Denver scenario is extreme, other examples exist. Rutter reports that Adrienne Anderson, an activist and a professor in the Environmental Studies Program and Ethnic Studies Department at the University of Colorado, uncovered (another) agreement that allows Lockheed Martin in Littleton, Colorado to pipe toxic wastes into the Littleton/Englewood wastewater plant. At the plant, the waste would be turned into, yes, "beneficial biosolids" and used for agricultural purposes in eastern Colorado. Concern is also mounting for the Salt Lake area in Utah that, like Denver, is surrounded by military installations and Superfund sites. Crop failures have also been reported in Washington State, and investigations conducted by Patty Martin, the former mayor of Quincy, Washington revealed that Cenex/Land 'O Lakes, a local fertilizer company, had been dumping a toxic slew of heavy metals, pesticides, and radioactive materials on nearby farmland. Martin also found that Cenex/Land 'O Lakes was also selling similar versions of the same stew as fertilizer. And they weren't the only ones doing it.(72)

These events which occurred in Washington State are described in greater detail in a book by Duff Wilson. Copies of this book are available from used book dealers at very modest cost, and a brief account or Wilson's nonfiction book can be reviewed on Wikipedia under the title "Fateful Harvest".

ALSO IN LIQUID FERTILIZER

The above information clearly illustrates how toxic waste can find its way into farmland by being added in a solid form derived from sludge and/or sewage. Further research into this matter disclosed that these toxins could also find their way into farmland from liquid fertilizers. For example, in 1993 a North American farmer complained to Bill Rutherford, a local natural agricultural products company owner, that his corn crop's roots were "growing up" i.e., above the ground. He suspected that the corn roots were trying to avoid exposure to something toxic in the soil. Based on this complaint, Rutherford, who also manufactures fertilizer, asked the farmer to bring in a sample of the liquid fertilizer that he had applied to his cornfield. Rutherford sent this sample to an analytical laboratory. This analysis which I had an opportunity to review revealed that aluminum was present at a concentration of over 2200 parts per million. The test also disclosed that there were lesser amounts of arsenic and cadmium.

HEAVY METAL MEALS

Along with aluminum, these metals are toxic to life and have no biologic value or worth. In March 2012, a representative from a government agency charged with regulating the content of fertilizers assured me that some farmland in the U.S. has a naturally high aluminum content. However, Jon Frank of International Ag Labs, Inc. cautioned that in high aluminum soils adequate calcium also needs to be present. And Rutherford noted in a conversation we had in May, 2012 that sulfur and selenium are present in very low levels in some North American farm soils, and that the presence of one pound of sulfur is required for every seven pounds of nitrogen for proper utilization of the nitrogen. He told me soil selenium is so low in his area that it has to be supplemented in triple the usual amount, a quantity so high that it requires a veterinarian's prescription. In the absence of adequate selenium he has witnessed the death of livestock, such as sows, from heart disease.

An information sheet distributed by the manufacturer of the liquid fertilizer in question noted that some of their products may undergo a color change due to the presence of "stray copper." This company's letter announced that they were working with their supplier to remove the copper. Rutherford told me that the presence of copper in the fertilizer raised the suspicion that industrial waste was being used as a filler. He draws his knowledge and experience from his firm's manufacturing of liquid minerals and plant food. He also noted that it was common practice for commercial liquid chemical fertilizers to contain spent (i.e. waste) phosphoric acid that was originally used in the cleaning or "pickling" process for the smelting of metal. He also told me that this form of phosphoric acid would not be biologically available to the crops until it was converted into usable ingredients by soil organisms. He pointed out that the conversion would only occur if the soil temperature were above 55 degrees F. He explained that this required temperature would not typically be reached in the soil in the spring rendering the essential ingredient of this fertilizer unusable at the time when it is applied and needed the most.

WILL THE TRUTH EVEN SURFACE?

A representative of the laboratory that analyzed the liquid fertilizer told me in summer, 2011 that agricultural soil analyses do not typically check for the presence of toxic metals and that determinations generally are made on soil samples only to a depth of six inches. I inquired of this representative what toxic metals might be residing in the subsoil after decades of being treated with fertilizer laden with hazardous industrial waste? His reply was "No one has ever looked there.".

FOR HOW MANY DECADES?

In 2001, the Seattle Times reported that the Washington Toxics Coalition and the Sierra Club had sued the EPA in 1998 for failing to regulate the amount of hazardous waste in fertilizers as aggressively as they did the hazardous waste in landfills. The primary issue that instigated the suit was the finding of heavy metals such as lead and cadmium, as well as dioxins, in fertilizers and the finding that these ingredients were derived from the "zinc dust" from recyclers' furnaces. A seemingly positive result of this lawsuit was that the states of Washington, California and Texas began to limit the heavy metal content of fertilizers, but there were many compromises in their regulations.(74)

MONITOR IT BUT DON'T STOP IT

For example, in Washington, full-disclosure labeling was mandated, but the effectiveness of this measure was lessened, because buyers of the fertilizer had to look on the Internet, not on the label attached to the bag itself, to find the disclosure information. And even more compromising, the same legislative act that mandated full disclosure labeling also legalized the practice of disposing of hazardous waste via fertilizer.(74) We must ask how the EPA could allow laws like this? In this situation, the EPA is "absolved from responsibility" because fertilizer regulation is relegated to the individual states.(74)

WHO KNOWS? WHO KNOWS?

Today, some fertilizer companies are not using hazardous waste as filler in their products. However, personal communication with one fertilizer industry representative left the author with the impression that this industry is not yet completely "whistle clean". I do not believe that the fertilizer industry will be completely free from this practice for three reasons. The first is that current laws allow hazardous waste to be included in fertilizers. The second is that using hazardous waste in fertilizer is profitable, and the third is that the public is largely unaware of how dangerous this practice is. Thus, what incentive is there to change?

IT KEEPS STACKING UP

So far, this chapter has primarily discussed the dangers to our farmland and our health because of dangerous and immoral hazardous waste disposal practices that allow poisons and toxins to be added to fertilizers. The remainder of this chapter will address the dangers of products that are used to treat our crops and soils, such as agricultural chemicals, sprays, insecticides, herbicides, and fungicides.

A PERSONNAL TESTIMONY

I became very aware of the dangers of products that were used to treat our crops and soils many years ago when I was part of a research team at Columbia University in New York. Our group investigated the toxicity of agricultural chemicals that were aerosolized inside an orchid green house by the owner who had developed a brain cancer which in quick order took his life. We discovered that one of the aerosolized chemicals, a fungicide, damaged the DNA (genes) of experimental animals that were exposed to it. Some of these animals developed pulmonary tumors. The exact mechanism of DNA damage was determined by sophisticated laboratory techniques and the results were published in a scientific journal.(75) This information has been accessible now for over 40 years. Nevertheless, this fungicide, captan, is still in wide use throughout the world. It is also incorporated into plastics, oil-based paints, textiles, paper, and cosmetics; and it is used as a mold- and mildew-proofing agent in coatings intended for contact with certain types of foods.(76)

A LARGE-SCALE PROBLEM

The foregoing example referred to scientific studies that revealed how a particular fungicide caused damage to DNA, the genetic material. This was the proposed or suspected mechanism whereby that particular agricultural chemical was able to cause a fatal cancer in a human being. Since we are exposed to a myriad environmental toxins including heavy metals, plastics, pesticides, industrial chemicals, and cancer-causing hydrocarbons, one might wonder what mechanisms allow these toxins to damage our health. In actuality, there are a number of ways through which various chemicals and toxins wreak their effect. Although it is not necessary to understand the nature of these mechanisms to grasp the message of this book, I think it will be helpful to the reader to provide a semi "in depth" presentation of how one representative agricultural product adversely affects living things.

1OO MILLION POUNDS

The illustrative agent that I will discuss in more detail is glyphosate which was mentioned earlier in this chapter. It is the active ingredient in a weed killer (herbicide) that is widely used in farms, yards, and parks throughout the world. As noted above, in the U.S. alone over 100 million pounds are applied yearly.(58)

EXTENSION

Many weed killers work by destroying certain enzymes needed for growth of the plant (or weed). Glyphosate specifically works by acting as a strong chelating agent after the plant absorbs it in the following fashion. Chelation here means this chemical product strongly binds to metallic ions and thus makes them unavailable to the plant that requires these good metals for its enzymes to be active and for other nutritional needs. This causes the plant to die.(58)

Glyphosate is an especially strong chelator of manganese, but also acts on zinc, copper, iron, and other metals. In fact, glyphosate was originally patented as a chelating agent in 1964. The use of glyphosate to get rid of weeds causes a problem because crop (i.e., food) plants can't use manganese in its oxidized form; it first has to be changed into its reduced form by soil organisms which themselves require manganese as a nutrient. The soil organisms suffer from the unavailability of manganese and the crops are also damaged for the same reason. Research has shown the magnitude of this problem by showing that after treatment with products containing glyphosate, entire groups of beneficial organisms are disappearing from the soil.(58)

SOON THEY WILL BE MINING HERBICIDE FROM THE FARM SOIL

After exposure to a glyphosate-containing herbicide, these

food plants grow poorly, and they are more susceptible to disease because this chemical also compromises the plant's resistance by inhibiting the plant's disease defense mechanisms. The glyphosate accumulates in the grain and roots soon after it is applied, and what doesn't get taken up by the plant can remain in the soil for as long as 22 years. For every four pounds of glyphosate applied to the soil, three pounds has been recovered in following years. In fact, the French Supreme Court ruled it was fraud for the manufacturer to claim that glyphosate was biodegradable. Chiseling (cutting deep into the soil with an implement) decreases its toxicity by increasing nutrient availability even though there may be little effect on its persistence.(58)

A LITTLE WON'T HURT YOU?

Since glyphosate accumulates in the grains, it enters the body when the absorbing plants such as corn, soybeans, or wheat are eaten. Can this be dangerous to our health? It would seem so because, although glyphosate is touted as safe by some agricultural agents, ingesting about one quarter of a cup of weed killer can be lethal.(58)

DO THE BENEFITS OUTWEIGH THE HARM DONE?

Glyphosate also decreases photosynthesis in food plants and crops, impairs nitrogen fixation, interferes with phosphate absorption, kills beneficial microbes, and, as noted above, reduces the growth and development of earthworms. It was also found that sterility and miscarriage developed in cattle that were fed feed from fields to which it had been applied. The mechanism of such action (which also causes infertility in pigs, sheep, and chicken) is that this herbicide disrupts normal endocrine hormone function, interferes with enzymes called aromatases, and predisposes plants to a new, highly toxic compound that increases the spontaneous abortion rate in farm animals. (58)

THIS HAS TO STOP

I have only mentioned a few of the problems in which products with glyphosate are suspected to have a role. There are other dangerous ingredients in weed killers as well. In fact, some, and perhaps many, of the adverse reactions that have been attributed to weed killers may be caused by dangerous additives the label hides –but does not list-- under the term of "other ingredients." One of these "ingredients", polyethoxylated tallowamine, or POEA, was the subject of recent experiments in France. These experiments revealed that POEA was deadly to human embryonic, placental, and umbilical cord cells. POEA was shown to be deadly to those cells in amounts far below agricultural recommendations and corresponding to the low levels of residue typically found in human food or animal feed. (57)

In an attempt to minimize the damage done by glyphosate, scientists developed a method of increasing tolerance of it by adding a gene conferring resistance to it that was harvested from a soil bacterium. However, only mature plants are protected by this method. Plants at the delicate, developing stage are still vulnerable.(58) And, as the evidence presented and referenced above suggests, tissues are most sensitive to toxins in the early stages of their development.

WILL WE BE THE LAST TO CHANGE?

Scientists, especially in Europe, are concerned because glyphosate-containing herbicides are being used on such a large scale with little or no regulation. They fear damaging amounts of this endocrine disrupter will poison our soil and our drinking water. As such, it has been predicted that its days in Europe are numbered.(58)

A VOICE CRYING OUT IN THE DARKNESS

Dr. Don Huber, Professor Emeritus from Purdue University, who has studied this particular herbicide extensively, has stated that we are on the precipice of a situation which threatens the sustainability of agriculture. He adds that no agricultural threat of the past compares with this threat and that symptoms of it have progressed, for the most part unrecognized, and certainly unaddressed, for 15-16 years and for these no "quick fix" exists.(58)

WILL ANYONE BE ALIVE TO WRITE THE FINAL REPORT?

In summary, glyphosate is one of the 2,863 chemicals that are produced in excess of one million pounds annually in this country, only 12 of which have been tested for neuro-developmental toxicity according to EPA guidelines.(52, 53) And we know that, at least with respect to toxic metals, that the damage resulting from exposure to multiple agents is not additive but multiplicative. (77) Critical research has not been done, so we can only ask what effect an ingredient like this has on the development of autism in our children and on the normal growth and development of all children? And what effects do all the other ingredients that are being used on our farmlands have on the development of autism and on the normal development of children?

HOLD ON! THERE IS HOPE

There must be a solution. And there is a solution. First, however, we will briefly review another dangerous practice that is affecting our food supply and the health of our children and ourselves. As a nation we are now consuming genetically modified (GM) foods in ever-increasing amounts. Is consuming genetically modified foods dangerous?

ANOTHER LARGE-SCALE PROBLEM

Tomatoes were the first crops where GM technology was used. When these tomatoes were introduced by tube into the stomach of rats, 7 of 40 animals died. Erosions and necrosis (death) of their internal stomach lining cells occurred. The GM tomatoes have since been withdrawn from the market. Genetically modified potatoes also damaged the gut when they were fed to experimental animals. These potatoes caused an increase in the number of a particular white blood cell (lymphocytes) in the intestinal wall that was similar to an increase that would be caused if an infection were present there. The gut wall thickness of these rats also increased by 50% in reaction to being fed the GM potatoes.(78)

IT'S JUST NOT NATURAL

Farmers in the Philippines working with GM corn developed runny noses, allergies, and wheezing. GM crops always evoke an immune response. Abnormal changes were seen in the liver and pancreas of mice fed GM soy. A small, but measurable, amount of GM DNA (genetic material) was found in the gut bacteria of human subjects. In another experiment, GM soy was fed to pregnant rats two weeks before lactation. The mothers and their pups in the control group (no GM food) were larger. There were fewer offspring in the treated group and in male animals the testicular size was smaller. This certainly could affect reproduction Similar abnormalities were encountered in mice fed GM corn.(78)

NO ONE IS WATCHING OUT FOR THE USA

The largest seed grower in Europe will not allow GM crops to be grown on its land. Europeans decline to eat GM food as do some domestic and wild animals and rodents. GM corn, soy, and potatoes have been surreptitiously introduced into our food chain and these foods were being ingested unbeknownst to the public for three years. In a recent presentation in Canada it was stated that the biotech companies that are creating GM food are not studying its effects on reproduction, cancer, allergies, the immune and hormonal systems, and on human beings.(78)

WHO KNOWS THE LONG-TERM EFFECTS?

It is true that the growth of some pests, such as aphids and nematodes, is decreased in GM crops, but so are some desirable species such as lady bugs. Finally, in the process of genetic modification, 4000-5000 genes (2-4% of the entire genetic makeup of the food being treated) also are being altered.(78)

We do not have all the answers on the safety of GM food at this time, and it will probably be years before our knowledge reaches a measure of sufficiency. However, there are many problems in our world where GM food enters the food chain of man or animals, and many experiments are pointing to the peril of consuming GM food. Recent study of urban Canadian women showed that 93% of the study sample contained GM corn toxin in their blood, and 80% passed this toxin to the developing child in their womb.(79) Because of these suspected or real dangers, Europe has banned them. And many other nations have followed suit. As mentioned above, many animals won't eat anything that is GM. Given this situation, the prudent approach seems to be to avoid consuming GM foods until their safety is proven. Meanwhile, the government of the United States should realize the dangers of GM foods and act to remove them from the marketplace. It is a good idea to avoid processed foods as the great majority of these contain GM foods or ingredients obtained from them.

PROFIT OVER HEALTH

GM food has been proven to be very unhealthy by numerous

experiments as well as by many life occurrences. Unfortunately the incentive for large companies to produce GM seeds is immense because of the monopoly that is produced for the seed and fertilizer companies. First of all, some seeds are infertile. This means farmers using them can no longer save the seeds from their current crops, a practice of farmers from time immemorial. Instead, the farmer must dig into his pocket to purchase new seeds each year. In addition, fertilizer companies also benefit because GM crops are intentionally modified to be resistant to certain pesticides. Therefore, the farmer must use a specific pesticide designed for that GM crop.

In summary, there are four reasons why the food that we normally consume may be dangerously unhealthy for our children and ourselves.

1) The food we of the Western world chose to eat predictably contains excessive amounts of highly processed substances such as white sugar, white flour, and white animal fat. Our insatiable demand for such fare fuels its ever greater production. To increase palatability --and therefore sales-- it is adulterated with chemical colors, counterfeit flavoring agents, texturizers, taste enhancers as MSG, preservatives, hormones used to produce rapid growth in animals, antibiotics, high fructose corn syrup, or artificial sweetening agents such as aspartame. This fake sweetener and MSG in foods are known to warp our neurotransmitters, the messengers of our thoughts. An important manifestation of such twisting of nature is hyperexcitable behavior. The chemical agents which induce such abnormal behavior are called excitotoxins Add to this long list the foreign proteins from genetic modification. It seems to me that the worst way to

ruin food is to shotgun it with genes from other species, including human DNA. Is this stuff still food?

2) Commercial food is clearly deficient in natural, essential nutrients due either to over-processing and/or to having been grown in grossly nutritionally depleted soil.

3) In addition, such food can contain dangerous chemicals and poisons from their residues in and on it following applications to prevent weeds and diseases in both plants and animals. These agricultural chemicals have been shown for 60 years to be poisonous to living things (not just to the targeted pest or disease).(61) They are also causing irreparable damage to our ecosystem as the U.N. Millennium Report and its 2006 Update warned. (52,65)

4) Additional harm to the food accrues because of the contaminants in fertilizer that were applied to our farmland. This dangerous and immoral practice of disposing of industrial waste and other poisons in fertilizer has been going on for decades, and I suspect that many farmers completely unaware that these fertilizers have been de-decreasing the crop yield and destroying their soil. This is partly due to the truth being distorted and diluted by the lust for a dollar in the serpentine chain of those responsible for the provision of these artificial and tainted amendments.

WHO KNOWS WHAT'S IN IT?

The indisputable conclusion from the foregoing is that our food is certainly not safe for mothers- to-be nor for consumption by children who have impaired means of removing toxins from their body, such as children suffering from autism and ADHD. In addition, modern commercial food such as ours cannot be recommended for consumption to any prospective parents who wish to avoid these disorders in their offspring. Finally, realizing what is happening with our food supply, the reader is left to speculate if such "food" should be eaten by anyone, for it is abundantly clear that people who consume our modern food are exposed to multitude of interrelated risks.

ORGANIC FOOD IS NOT PERFECT

Faced with facts as these, can anyone doubt that at least some poisons and toxins find their way into modernly grown food, and then into the bodies of people consuming that food? Where does this leave the typical consumers who purchase their food in a grocery store? How could they possibly determine whether or not the food that they purchase was subjected to toxins during its growing and processing? This is such an immense problem that, if you are dealing with an immune-compromised individual like a child with autism who is unusually sensitive to environmental toxins, it would be better not to take the chance and to purchase fresh, organic, non-processed food instead. However, there are three drawbacks to this practice.

The first is that organically grown foods costs more, so much more in some areas, in fact, that this expense would be beyond the means of many.

The second drawback is that there is no assurance that organically grown foods were not grown in soil that had been receiving doses of toxic fertilizer if the farm was recently converted to grow organic crops. The certification process that allows food grown organically to be labeled as such requires only three years of artificial chemical-free farming. However, what had been accumulating in the soil over decades and is still resident there could certainly be assimilated (incorporated) into the organic crops. In support of this risk is the work of Rachel Carson who noted that some food crops as carrots actually concentrate pesticides to levels greater than those found in the soil in which they were grown. (61)

The final drawback relates to the common practices of organic food growers. Yes, most food certified to be organically grown is quite likely to be free of noxious chemicals, but may still be lacking in nutrients, the addition of which to any farm soil can be expensive and decrease the margin of profit.

THE LESSON ON TWO LEVELS

We will make the point later in this book that, for persons trapped in our cities, the only alternative is to purchase organic food. I sincerely believe that this practice will provide important health benefits, subject to the limitations noted above.

EVEN WITH ORGANIC FOODS SUPPLEMENTS WILL ALWAYS BE NEEDED

In the book, Super Nutrition Gardening, two agricultural scientists write that a plant, including a food plant, requires 17 minerals, but that the human body requires 23.(80) This means that the organic food that we purchase may be pure and even perfectly healthy, but nevertheless insufficient in minerals such as selenium and iodine to make it nutritionally complete for humans. As noted, it is expensive to amend the soil and the soil analyses performed at state agricultural laboratories do not check for the presence of many essential nutrients. A laboratory exists that will test a soil sample for all the required nutrients and make recommendations for what specific nutrients must be added to that soil to make it complete.(73) However, the cost of spreading these nutrients over acres of farmland would be very expensive. It would also be impossible for every family with a child suffering from autism to move to a traditional farm.

WHAT'S NEXT?

What, then, remains? What can be done short of every family with a child suffering from autism moving to a standard farm where such nutrients could be added? What is the answer to this modern dilemma?

The Solution

THE FACTS ARE THE FACTS

The reader can conclude from the above material that we live in a very toxic and poisonous world and that our children, especially those with ASDs, suffer greatly from this. Respected scientists soberly warn us that something must be done if the human race is to survive. (52,65) Based on past and present experiences we cannot rely on our government, factory farming, or on big industry to solve the myriad of problems that we face since they have a history of taking advantage of the little guy, in this case the farmer and his land. Either this smaller grower is unaware of their doings or he is unable to raise the funds to fight them in court and win. Clearly, the situation is out of hand. Our environment has already become too damaged for any currently mandated regulations to reverse and remedy.

THE SURE WAY TO HELP

The only reasonable solution remaining is to take the matter of food production into our own hands. This is a splendid way to ensure pure, fresh, safe, and nutritionally complete food for our families. The crux of the matter is that the father of a family, whom God by natural law has designated as its protector and provider, should not delegate or surrender the safety of his family's food supply to anyone.

Instead, the father of a family at this time in our history should strive his utmost to gain control over what his family eats by growing and raising it on the family's own small piece of land. This measure is needed now because "the system" has made the food supply unsafe. Sad but true, we live in a period of history when the lust for the dollar dominates nearly every secular organization and corporation; and "good old boy politics" often rule government and business deals. In such a tainted setting, commercially offered chemical "edibles" can only reflect the conditions under which they were created.

AN INTERESTING AND IMPORTANT FACT

There is an amazing additional benefit that raising crops in one's own naturally cared-for soil provides. The numerous microorganisms present in such soil have the capability of indirectly nullifying the deleterious effect of radioactivity. (I will explain why the benefit is an indirect one). Two agricultural researchers from Peuerbach, Austria discovered that microbes accomplish this negation of damage by radioactivity in their book *Pioneers of Controlled Microbial Composting*. These scientists were using natural methods, including microbially inoculated, humus-rich compost, on their organic farm located downwind from the Chernoble nuclear plant in Russia. The terrible meltdown in this facility released a large amount of radioactive heavy metals into the air which settled on the ground both in and around their farm fields. To their surprise, the humus-rich soil, despite being saturated with fallout from a contaminating nuclear cloud, somehow, with the help of all its microorganisms, supported growth of a root vegetable crop devoid of radioactivity.(81) In Peuerbach, the presence of radioactive contamination indicated the presence of heavy metals, and the metal toxicity was worse because these metals in addition were radioactive.

This is particularly noteworthy because the radiation was detectable in the root vegetables grown in the soil of surrounding farms that were not rich in the humus matter derived from composted manure.

GOOD SOIL VS RADIOACTIVITY

The radioactive contaminants produced by the Chernoble accident and that settled on the soil included the metal caesium. Research reveals that metals in the soil, lead and cadmium (which have no business being there), are absorbed by potatoes in increased concentration in a range that the content of these metals in the tubers was several times higher than the limit value. (82). Carrots have been shown to concentrate harmful pesticides threefold greater than is present in the surrounding soil. (61). However, organic soil additives (peat, compost, and vermacompost) effectively immobilized lead, copper, zinc, and cadmium in the soil in the vicinity of a smelting operation and decreased their uptake by potato plants growing in that soil. Such use of organic soil amendments and agronomic practices is called phytoremediation. (83) This process of humus management, which removes pollutants from the environment or decreases their toxicity, may explain the unique lack of detectable radioactivity in root vegetable crops grown downwind from the Chernoble nuclear accident.

WHAT PROOF DO WE NEED?

Recalling that this book is devoted to the prevention, management, and care of autism, I return to my interview with a member of the Amish community mentioned near the end of Chapter Two. I spoke with a farmer who told me that some Amish people allow their children to be vaccinated, but this usually doesn't occur before the age of two years. Also, it is common practice to spread the immunizations out over time. This man corroborated the observation that autism is extremely rare among the Amish. He told me that, for the most part, the Amish people's food supply comes from the crops they produce on their own naturally fertilized land, and that their source of meat is the animals they raise. Such food is fresh, pure, and nutrient-dense. It would be hard to determine if the relaxed vaccination schedule, the healthy country environment with home-grown food, or even a strong and spiritual family life prevent autism from developing in Amish communities. It is most likely a combination of all these. I believe that the excellent condition of the soil on Amish farms plays a major role in the low autism rate they experience.

THIS IS REALLY POSITIVE NEWS!

Another compelling example of the importance of naturally healthy farm soil in preventing the development of autism is the current experience in Cuba. The needed inflow of Russian chemical fertilizer halted with the U.S. embargo and with the collapse of the Soviet Bloc, leaving Cuba to develop alternative measures. The government wisely turned to vermacomposting, a means of naturally caring for the soil. Twenty years ago there were already 172 centers distributed throughout Cuba using this technology. In these operations one can see firsthand a bountiful harvest of long windrows of red earthworm casings resulting from large-scale conversion of animal manure and other organic waste into the finest of all natural fertilizers. (84) Earthworms manufacture humus, the vital, nutrient-rich, porous, moisture-holding component of topsoil. The production of humus is the most critical contributor to the natural care of the soil. (85)

The amazing situation is that, despite a rigorous vaccination schedule and a high immunization compliance rate, autism rarely develops in Cuba. The incidence there is 0.00168% versus a U.S. incidence of 0.50%. In other words the US autism rate is 298 x's that in Cuba (86) Contrast Cuba's autism rate to the extremely high incidence of autism in Romania (71), another Communist country, where the environment is deplorably damaged (70) and, we presume, the use of artificial fertilizer is widespread.

THERE IS A WAY OUT

A family with a child struggling with autism has a special need to live on the land and be in control of its own food supply. This fact should be obvious after reading the above discouraging words about our country's poor quality, store-bought food. This being the case, one may ask "What can be done and how?" In answer, I will now attempt to describe a means to accomplish this.

SEEK THE PROPER LOCATION

Families must live in areas of the country where they can plant gardens and keep animals. First, a family must agree to adopt such a lifestyle in order to gain adequate control of its food supply. The next step is to hopefully find property that has not been used as farmland in the past, in other words, land that has not been heavily artificially fertilized. Such land should be located in an area where both air and water are not also heavily chemically contaminated. As has been mentioned, nearly any soil can be renewed and purified with the proper care. However, time, effort, and sometimes years are needed in order to restore the land to the best quality. Therefore, finding unspoiled land is the best way to go. Locating such a parcel is not as difficult as it may seem, since small acreage packages still exist that surrounding features or topography have rendered unsuitable for cultivation by modern day agricultural equipment.

A PLAN FOR THE PROPERTY

After the piece of property has been selected, the next step is to prepare a plan for its proper use. Reasons for such needed forethought include a garden's need to have as much sunshine as possible. Also, the barn should be located downwind from the living quarters of the family. Other considerations are the positioning of the driveway and how the land should drain. If necessary, a civil engineer can be hired to prepare a proposal for the particular property chosen. He may direct a surveyor to construct a topographical map of the land which will be invaluable for future planning and applications for permits. In order to become better acquainted with such planning aids much additional information is available from organizations using the term "permaculture".

GET EDUCATED

After a plan has been prepared and finalized, studies can be undertaken related to building a garden and animal facilities. The garden is really central to having full control of a family's food supply. Milk, eggs, meat, and, most importantly, a constant supply of natural fertilizer are also necessary. This can only be accomplished by having both a garden and a barn or other suitable shelters for animals and fowl. Magazines and books abound from which a family can learn how to construct and operate such improvements to the land. One only needs to tie into this information network.

BUILD TO LAST

All must be done in a way to ensure endurance. Constructing a garden with permanent raised beds will make it easier to grow crops and to maintain the garden for untold decades. The same applies to all the animal and fowl facilities. Think of such improvements to the land as one would think of a house. Most people do not build a temporary shelter in which to live. Instead, they do the best job they possibly can in its planning and construction. This line of thinking must also rule when building a garden and a barn. Such an approach is well-justified. For, once up and running, these facilities will provide all the food for the family for the rest of their lives.

A LASTING SOURCE

Of course, the need to go to the health foods store to obtain salt, spices, or other products that cannot be gown in one's part of the country will continue, but such purchases will be minimal. The bulk of a family's food supply can be grown or produced on the land a family owns. This is the natural way to provide what the family eats. Such has been the case since the very beginning. Our Creator intended it this way. This becomes obvious to anyone who has ever had a garden or kept animals. This plan is the best way to ensure a constant source of food for one's family, sustenance that is fresh, pure and nutritious. It is nothing short of a necessity for all children with autism, and it is really what is best for all human beings. It is difficult to effectively refute this point.

HEALTHY BODIES

Living this type of lifestyle has other health benefits. Most importantly, it means the family members have to do some simple, manual labor daily. In essence, they have to exercise to eat. Really, this is best for everyone. Our bodies were made to be used. Without exercise we suffer from poor digestion and we do not have strong muscles, nor can the skeletal portions of our body be kept in order. Having to work to eat simply means that working is a necessity. The physical fitness needed to accomplish this is essential to the health of every able family member. Those less able should be encouraged and expected to contribute whatever they can to this vital domestic effort.

FAMILY UNION ALSO

Living this lifestyle naturally brings all household members together frequently for a number of activities, for everyone must learn to work as a team to meet the family's needs. The result is a growing love among the parents and children, plentiful caring and sharing, and a good measure of giving and sacrifice. What a contrast this way of living is compared with the way most people live in today's world! Reflect a moment on how changing to family gardening and the raising of smaller animals is a change for the better. It is a very positive move that all family members can, and should, embrace with enthusiasm.

WHAT TO GROW; WHAT TO RAISE

The food crops can be selected and grown based on their nutritional value and in accordance with the recommendations set forth in Dr. Cabot's books, as will be discussed in Chapter Six. The animals should include goats, sheep, and rabbits. A family also needs chickens for the eggs they provide. But large animals should be avoided since they are dangerous. Horses and cows can injure a person just by stepping on one's foot.

DON'T BE STUBBORN

Perhaps, the only other animals to consider raising are donkeys. They are lovable creatures, come in all sizes, and are excellent for protecting sheep and goats from predators. Although they may be considered extra to the plan, they are justified because of the demonstrated positive effect animals have on children with autism, as our experience with them readily demonstrates.

ULTIMATE SECURITY

A family could also keep and raise earthworms on a large scale. The benefits to the soil are tremendous. These advantages are again noted in the chapter that follows. Implementing this measure and all else recommended above can ensure a family has the best food possible, food that meets the nutritional requirements to enable a child with autism to lead a personally tolerable life, one that is agreeable to his or her family members, and a life as productive as potential permits.

Without adopting the above lifestyle, the security and safety of the food supply will always be in question, as the material presented earlier in this chapter so clearly demonstrates.

A drastic measure, you may think, an extreme one? Yes, initially it may seem so. But in truth no other lifestyle can begin to compare with it. Why? The answer lies in the acute sensitivity a child with autism exhibits to anything entering the body by whatever route. Natural living minimizes these detrimental exposures. In addition, a child with autism reaps undeniable benefits from contact with affectionate animals. This remarkable finding and other equally fascinating facts are explored further in the next chapter.

ROLL UP YOUR SLEEVES AND GET THE JOB DONE

In conclusion, hope abounds for the child with autism and his or her family, although the skies are indeed dark and our water can be extremely dirty. That hope materializes when a family takes the route to become independent of the system's food supply and enjoy the numerous other benefits noted above.

Such a healthy way of living can happen for your family, your child, and you. Just add determination, effort, and action. This means getting focused and getting going, for time is a relentless, unforgiving enemy.

This is my firm recommendation.

Chapter Five

Help From The Barn

The Problem

IMPORTANCE OF SOIL FERTILITY

On the eve of WWII, a British agricultural scientist, Sir Albert Howard, wrote a book in which he analyzed the agricultural practices of civilizations that survived the test of time, as well as the practices of those which did not. Howard reached the remarkable conclusion that whole civilizations have passed out of existence simply because their soil was infertile. He described the cultivated soil as the real capital [currency] of the nations, observing that the decay of past civilizations occurred because of the decline in soil fertility. He emphasized that our own civilization was endangered for this very same reason. However, Howard ended his book on a hopeful note. The situation can be saved, he wrote, if people could only be convinced of the vital connection that exists between fertile soil and healthy crops, healthy animals, and healthy humans. Howard felt strongly that persons raised in a society with fertile soil would be normal and vigorous human beings and achieve the highest degree of physical and mental development. (85)

DOUBLE PROBLEM

In support of Howard's contention just prior to WWII, the then U.S. Secretary of Agriculture lamented that man treats nature harshly. He stated that man overplows the cropland and eventually destroys the soil. (59) In the interval since WWII, the situation has only worsened. Today, the soil is not only infertile but also toxic. This book is raising "red flags" about the safety of our food supply. We have multiple problems. What we are eating everyday not only lacks essential nutrients, but it is also laden with both harmful agricultural chemicals and extremely toxic industrial waste, which has been used as a filler in both solid and liquid artificial fertilizers.

NATURE'S ROUND

This is where my investigation into the cause and treatment of autism has led. What is going on? What has gone wrong, and why? The solution to this modern catastrophe requires an understanding of what comprises the soil and how the Creator has woven a major fiber into the fabric of the survival garment of all species. This fiber is an endless resilient thread that Sir Howard calls "nature's round". It is the orderly evolution of the wheel of life. It results from the adoption and execution of the first principle of agriculture. This principle states that there must always be a perfect balance between the processes of growth and decay. The wonderful consequences of this perfect balance are a living soil, abundant good crops, and higher species, including man, who enjoy great health. (85)

NEED LIFE TO SUPPORT LIFE

Unfortunately, our agriculture has become unbalanced, and diseases of all kinds are on the increase. Too much attention has been paid to forcing the land to produce crops year after year without giving heed to what Howard terms the "manurial" rights of the soil. The lesson we have learned all too poorly is the impossibility of replacing manure from animals with any man-made substance. Man-made fertilizers are dead. On the other hand, manure teems with life, the life that is needed to complete nature's cycle of life. (85) The tiny microorganisms which comprise 30% of animal manure are just as vital a part of the farmer's livestock as are barnyard animals, and they require equal care and attention. Both forms of livestock, creatures both large and small, have a vital part to play in keeping farms and gardens healthy. There is no other way. Why?

The Solution

IMORTANT ROLE OF DOMESTIC ANIMALS

Life begins in the soil and ends in the soil in a cycle of life that will never change. Plant life begins and continues in the soil because the soil contains what each plant requires: food for growth and development. The surrounding air and water in the soil also contribute some nourishment. For the sake of simplicity and to make the matter understandable, this chapter addresses the nourishment supplied by the soil. The essential role of domestic animals in this process and how they contribute to maintaining our mental and physical health will become quite evident.

IMPORTANCE OF SOIL LIFE

In order for the soil to nourish plants, it has to be full of little living creatures, the presence of which in earthen material is the difference between living soil and plain, old, dead dirt. These little creatures in the soil --call them friendly or helpful microbes-- are too small to be seen with the naked eye, but what they achieve is nothing short of miraculous. They convert small particles of rock or sand, granules of minerals, and organic matter into even smaller particles, tiny enough that a plant root then somehow absorbs them to nourish the plant and fuel its growth. The survival of the plant depends on the presence and activity of these myriad microscopic creatures in the soil. Without them the plant would not be able to produce leaves, seeds, fruit, or any other plant material that animals and humans alike require for their own survival.

IMPORTANCE OF NATURAL FERTILIZER

Realization of this basic principle enables a person or a family to understand why the presence of animals in the schema is essential for they provide food for these soil creatures in order that the whole food growing process can operate. They make it possible for a person or a family to to cultivate a garden, plant a field of grain, or grow trees for their bounty of fruits and nuts. The presence of animal and fowl manure in the soil allows soil creatures to thrive and thereby nourish the plants. With the constant supply of manure and the passage of time, the soil becomes so enriched with plant food that it is able to support garden crops of all types, year in and year out. These crops have all the nutrients they need to grow into healthy, strong plants, full of goodness for the animals and people who will consume them. With healthy food the creatures and the human beings can also become healthy and strong, and hopefully, in the case of humans, also full of goodness. It is all natural. It is the best way.

IMPORTANCE OF MINERALS

The endless nurturing of the life in the soil is essential to the whole process of growing gardens and grains. As noted above, mineral particles must also be available. These comprise very many elements, all of them needed for plant growth and for the nourishment of higher species which live on them. When the soil is replete with these mineral elements and with the organic matter of which we will speak, including the panoply of little living creatures it needs to digest the earthen material, then everything that is required by vegetable and field crops is present and their nutrient needs are completely met.

HEALTHY PLANTS RESIST INSECTS

It is critical to note that if crops are provided with everything required to grow well they will also be healthy enough to resist attacks by insects because such plant enemies and diseases seek out only weak or unhealthy plants. This is a great, natural truth. The corollary is that such a condition of crop wellness averts the need for chemical insecticides.

IT'S NATURAL LAW

Such soil management is the underlying principle of "Organic" gardening. The natural approach keeps food pure and healthy. The man who originated the term "Organic," reiterated what he learned from Sir Albert Howard's work, namely, that "healthy soil results in healthy plants which results in healthy animals and in healthy people." (85) This concept captures what natural gardening care achieves.

KEEP SOIL HEALTHY

The vital principal is that all life begins in the soil. Once a person or a family grasps and accepts this truth they can take every means to ensure a healthy soil. They can act to provide the soil with the needed supplement of natural minerals, mostly from sea products, and sufficiently composted manure --ingredients every plant needs to be healthy and strong.

VERY INTERESTING

Amazingly, the life process which takes place inside of each of us is not unlike the above. True, we aren't kept alive by tiny pieces of rock, sand, or other particles. Instead, we thrive on vegetables, crops, the food products from animals and the processing of this food that occurs in our gastrointestinal tracts. The intestinal part, or gut as it sometimes called, is populated by billions and billions of tiny living creatures. These microbes comprise our intestinal microscopic flora which in a natural symbiotic relationship process the food we eat into a form our cells can use.

OUR VERY LITTLE HELPERS

For example, when presented with a fragment of potato or tomato, our flora digests it into a material form our body can recognize as food, then absorb, and finally assimilate. Without this tiny form of microscopic life in our intestines we would starve and lose our own lives. Enzymes are necessary adjuncts to this process. The point is that our bodies require not only food by mouth but also the presence of a resident flora in our gastrointestinal tracts. These microscopic flora transform the food which enters our intestines into nutrients which can then sustain life in our cells.

WE MUST CARE FOR OUR VERY LITTLE HELPERS

Understanding the above should motivate us to carefully maintain the living creatures who work within and for us. Supplements called probiotics and prebiotics (which nurture the probiotic organisms) help prevent takeover and replacement of the healthy flora by harmful microbial strains. These supplements are part of the care and support we must at times provide. But there is more: it is imperative we avoid ingesting many man-made chemicals, regardless of how innocuous they are touted to be. Our intestinal creatures not only cannot digest such foreign agents but they also cannot remain alive in the presence of this enemy within us, as was addressed in a previous chapter.

ANIMALS PROVIDE NATURAL FERTILIZER

To recapitulate and clarify, the soil demands the life that comes from animal waste. It is what Sir Howard called the soil's "manurial rights". (85) Otherwise, it would be impossible for the soil's army to digest all the mineral matter already present and which continues to find its way down from the surface of the ground. Thus, a person or family finds justification in keeping their own animals in order to provide a constant source of manure for the garden and field soil. These animals, as stated above, are not gangly, bestial giants. Two men can lift any of them into the back of a pickup truck. Nearly without exception, they are extremely friendly and gentle and they produce manure that is inoffensive and easy to handle. They are also not unlike us in their need to be fed nutritious food so they in turn can produce "food" similarly nutritious and beneficial for the little creatures in the soil working "down there beneath our feet" where all life begins.

ANIMALS PROVIDE ORGANIC MATTER

Animal waste also contains organic matter that the soil needs to produce plant food. Plant growth and subsequent harvesting deplete the soil of both mineral matter and organic material. Thus, it must be replenished with what it has given up or the whole process will grind to a halt. This is what happened in the United States just before WWII when only 39% of our cropland became commercially farmable. (59) All the rest had been lost to erosion because we had forgotten about nature's round (cycle), the need to balance the processes of nutrient removal and nutrient replenishment.

A WAY TO TELL HOW NUTRITIOUS CROPS ARE

In our food markets vegetables and fruits should be sold not by the pound but by their nutrient content. The latter can be estimated by a device called a Brix refractometer which measures mineral content of the produce. It costs about $100. (87) In fact, shoppers can now be seen in the produce section of stores measuring the Brix number of their prospective purchases. Imagine a world in which the produce offered is accompanied by a placard displaying an analysis of the soil in which it was grown. Wine connoisseurs typically know much more about the vineyard from which they procure their wine than the rest of us know about the farm from which we obtain our life-sustaining food.

RESOURCES

The interested reader can learn more about this subject of soil fertility and organic gardening in books written by J.J. Rodale, the founder of the organic movement in this country. I would also strongly recommend the excellent work by Sir Albert Howard entitled *An Agricultural Testament*. (85) Numerous organic gardening and natural farming magazines are also available and very helpful in many ways to organic gardeners and natural farmers.

A VICIOUS CIRCLE

These books and magazines also clearly show that bypassing the natural process and replacing animal manure with artificial chemical fertilizers both starves and poisons the soil. Such farming practices produce sick plants, sick animals, and sick humans.(85) One could imagine that some pharmaceutical firms produce medicines to treat illnesses caused by the use of chemicals made by one of their other divisions.

A RIGHT WAY, A WRONG WAY

In growing food it would be a great error not to understand the proper use and preparation of animal manure. Storing it in a huge heap called a manure pile quickly depletes it of its essential nitrogen, and spreading raw manure on a growing crop, especially one near harvest, is equally wrong. The manure must be left in the soil for many months before the garden crops are grown. Alternatively, it can be placed in a compost bin and left there for months until it is ready to be used as natural fertilizer. Periodic turning of the compost (for aeration) may shorten the process somewhat.

THE BEST WAY

A third, very effective way involves feeding the manure to a large quantity of earthworms in a defined space. The earthworms rapidly convert the animal waste into humus which is then added to the garden soil. This process is the ultimate, natural care of the soil. As noted above, Cuba has been using this process on a national scale because of the loss of a fertilizer supply after the breakdown of the Soviet Bloc. The good news is that Cuba has now gained almost complete independence from artificial fertilizer and imported pesticides as well. Cubans now process animal manure by this method for use on most, if not all, of its farm crops.(84) We can assume the great improvement in its national health and the subsequent low incidence of autism that was reported in ref. (86) are due to the implementation of this natural method of farming.

CAN'T ARGUE WITH THE RESULT

We believe that natural care and support of the soil and the food grown in it nurtures a child's body sufficiently to permit its toleration of a huge vaccination load without becoming ill. This belief infers that children in Cuba are being protected from developing autism because of the luxuriant, humus-rich farm soil on which the food is grown. In addition, the plenitude of soil organisms resulting from such healthy farming practices may have allowed healthy crops to grow in Cuba despite any remaining soil contaminants from the Russian fertilizer, just as healthy organisms in organic soil allowed root crops in an Austrian farm to grow free from hazardous contamination after the farmland had been exposed to radioactive heavy metal fallout from the Cherbonyl accident. (81)

LET'S DO SOME TESTING

To validate this stance, we recommend that a comparison be made of the concentration of contaminants in the soils and crops from Cuba and those from the State of California. The rationale behind this suggestion is the finding by Rachel Carson who wrote fifty years ago of widespread pesticide contamination of food. (88) Since then, with the avalanche of chemical agents and industrial waste that has been deposited on our farm soil, the toxicity of the ground in which our food is grown can only have worsened.

AN ADDITIONAL BENEFIT

Also, as earthworm populations under this natural method can double every 60-90 days, those worms not used to seed new compost piles are dried and used as supplemental protein for animals. Since this practice is sufficiently widespread in Cuba, an important health benefit might accrue to us. Earthworms are high in protein and contain the amino acid methionine, which is absent from seed grains. (89) Methionine is an essential component of our biochemical methylation cycle that is so important and oftentimes so defective in autism. This surfeit of methionine works its way up the food chain and, by enhancing the Cuban diet, may contribute to that country's low autism rate. This being the case, the methionine content in the food chain should be less in countries that primarily use grain to feed livestock, and thus contribute to a higher incidence of autism in these nations. Comparison of the methionine content of soil and the food grown in it produced by these two methods of agriculture should be a simple matter. Such data may already exist.

RETURN TO NATURAL LAW

Using the Cuba experience as a model, the whole world can enjoy a ray of hope that the days of chemical agriculture are numbered. Even the artificial fertilizer companies could survive the change by specializing in natural mineral amendments.

IT IS WHAT IS BEST

The purpose of this book is to discuss and investigate the causes, management, and prevention of autism. Thus, it cannot explain to any sufficient degree how to garden or care for animals. Other books are available to provide this information. What this book does hope to achieve, however, is to show that anyone can do what is required to have a garden or to keep animals. It is as natural as life itself! It is not only the way life began on this earth, it is the only way healthy life can continue. As such, keeping animals is simply "a must" in order that a person or family can have a constant supply of animal products to feed and nourish the life in the soil. This is the way it has always been and the way it must always be. It's obvious. It's inescapable. It has to happen, and the sooner it does happen, the better for all humankind and especially for our children and future children.

HEALTH FOR HEALTHY PEOPLE

Keeping and caring for domestic animals in this little Eden also ensures an ongoing supply of food products from the animals and fowl themselves. Home grown foods, such as goat's milk, eggs from domestic fowl, and meat from goats, sheep, chickens, or rabbits are fresh, pure, and nutrient-dense. They are also free from antibiotics, hormones, pesticides, toxins, and the contaminating conditions after harvesting. Who knows what has been done to our foods, where, or how this has occurred between their harvesting from unhealthy factory farms and our opening a can or package to eat them? Garden fresh food is a treasured ticket to the state of a healthy mind in a healthy body for all persons and families who have seen the light and acted on it.

SOMEBODY IS BEHIND ALL THIS

The light we speak of shines forth from the Source of all light and love. This love has been poured from the day of creation, not only into us, but also into these smaller domestic animals. They are so easy to care for and love. They quickly become a part of our personal or family country life. They were created to be dependent on us. They are happy and content to be living in barns on small pieces of property. They bond very well with adults and children. This bond produces a wonderful, natural, elating, enlivening substance. This bond and this substance, another gift from the life in the barn, comprise the final part of this chapter.

CHILDREN LOVE ANIMALS

My experience raising animals such as sheep, goats, and miniature donkeys has been very positive. Families frequently drop by so their children can play with them and pet them. A marketing survey by a well known fast food chain investigating sales incentives revealed that 80% of the time young children's dreams are about animals.(90) I suppose you can fabricate give-away plastic toys that make animal-like sounds, but these shams are just not like the real thing. For example, when Rosie, our two year old lamb, began to bleat distressfully, my wife and I rushed from opposite directions to find she had crawled through a hole in the fence and gotten separated from her mother. In a joyful few minutes, Rosie was shepherded back to her mother's side and the crisis was over. In events such as these my wife and I have grown close to our animals, and closer to one another.

ANIMALS HELP PEOPLE TO LAUGH AND LOVE

Animals certainly provide material for talk around the dinner table. They can keep the family in stitches laughing. For example, they sometimes become complete liars in order to get a second throw of hay or dish of grain. If one of us inquires whether they the have already been fed, they universally reply with a loud and definitive "No-o-o-o-o-o!". The birth of a new animal also brings the family together in the barn, especially in the collective effort to nurture a weak baby lamb or goat kid in order to help it survive. It's obvious that God made us with a natural desire that is fulfilled when we are around animals.

ANIMALS ARE AFFECTIONATE

Certain animals like being close to people, compared to other animals that run away when people approach. For example, goats are so friendly that they will follow you everywhere. Our ram relishes having his wooly head cradled in my arms in a time of silent bonding. Mr. Duffy, one of our floppy-eared rabbits, recently allowed himself to be held by children all day long at a recent Animal Assisted Therapy Day and preferred this attention, even to eating. (91) Just this morning, I felt the lick of his tiny tongue on the tip of my nose. And Rico, our cat, alerted by the sound of the motor, waits in the driveway for us to return from town to our family garden farm. Then he jumps up into our laps for a short ride down to the barn, purring contentedly while fanning out his paws.

AUTISM AND EQUESTRIAN THERAPY

The Animal Assisted Therapy Day mentioned above was held at a local ranch dedicated to the parallel process of rescue, rehabilitation, and restoration of humans and horses. Here, in a very spiritual atmosphere volunteers and trained professionals, working in community, have rehabilitated nearly a dozen horses from various circumstances. These steeds are of different size, color, and breed, and yet all respond incredibly well to kindly caring by allowing themselves to be used in the therapy of patients, including children with autism. I witnessed the trust and bonding that develops during this therapy in a little boy with autism who, escorted on either side by parent and therapist, passed silently before me as he calmly rode the horse, sitting in the saddle *facing backwards.* (91)

A GREAT SUCCESS STORY

In this context, it's important to mention that the university professor, Temple Grandin, overcame autism with the help of the animals that she loved and provided for so well. An inspirational movie has been made about her life and bearing her name. Her illness prevented her from speaking until she was four years old. Thus, she developed a great love and attachment for animals at a small farm. Today she has a doctorate and is a professor at Colorado State University. She is known both for her squeeze box, a form of autism therapy now commercially available, and also for contributing greatly to the humane treatment of animals, even those destined for slaughter, because she was able to appreciate what the animals were feeling. Dr. Grandin speaks nationally about her own

experience and healing.
Her website is www.templegrandin.com.

GREAT BENEFIT FOR CHILDREN

It is insufficient to visit animals once in a while. People interested in benefiting from them should keep them. Children experiencing what has to be done to raise animals, including all the inconvenience and self-sacrifice it sometimes entails, develop good work habits and self-discipline that are important in life. In other words, God uses the children's love of animals to teach them to deny themselves and acquire virtues, such as patience and gentleness.

THE ANIMAL-HUMAN BRAIN-GUT CONNECTION

Meg Olmert authored a remarkable book entitled *Made for Each Other.* In it she investigates the biological nature of the bond that forms between humans and animals and how this is mediated by the hormone oxytocin.(51) Her findings fit hand-in-glove with those of Dr. Martha Welch whose laboratory at Columbia University in New York has demonstrated how the continuous administration of oxytocin simultaneously heals both the intestine and the brain of experimental animals in whom inflammatory bowel disease has been induced.(50) The need for continuous administration of oxytocin to achieve healing in Welch's laboratory animals underscores the need for animals to be constantly tended on the land in order to achieve similar benefits. Sorry, even frequent trips to the zoo won't work nearly as well as the close nurturing of a family animal. Dogs don't fill the bill very well because they are not a contributing part of the food chain and natural care of the garden soil.

LOVE IS CONTAGIOUS

We find that the hearts of the parents of the children with autism who visit our little garden of paradise are oftentimes more deeply touched by their contact with loving animals than their children. Perhaps a situation of sustained contact with animals might also help parents, and especially mothers, to become better nurturers --and better healers.

A DIFFERENT SPECIALTY

The following paragraphs paraphrase and quote what Meg Olmert has written in her book. She notes that some animals have an extraordinary way with people. And there are people who have extraordinary ways with animals. (51) Saint Francis of Assisi was one such person who had a marvelous way with animals. He was well known for taming a savage wolf that was terrorizing a town in Italy.

THERE IS PROOF

Dr. Aaron Katcher, a psychiatrist at the Devereux Foundation in Glenmore, PA took a group of boys with severe ADHD and behavioral problems and paired them with rabbits, turtles, gerbils, and doves. He found that the presence of these creatures made the boys calmer and more attentive. Caring for animals helped them hear what others had to say. Katcher also found that interactions with animals lowered blood pressure and heart rate. (51)

THE SOCIAL HORMONE

In 1993, the *New York Times* featured an article on the hormone oxytocin which is responsible for labor contractions (the prescription form of it is called Pitocin) and milk ejection. The article reported that in animals oxytocin increased monogamous social bonds and parental devotion. In other words, oxytocin had the same effect for animal mothers that Katcher found occurred in his boys. (51)

THE WONDER OF IT ALL

Caring for animals releases oxytocin in humans and is

proposed to be the chemical behind the animal-human bond, and the main biological ingredient of domestication (51). In 2003, two South African researchers measured oxytocin levels in humans and dogs before, during, and after friendly interactions and found that oxytocin levels almost doubled in both the people and the dogs, making pets one of the most potent triggers of oxytocin levels in humans. Gentle human touch can also decrease levels of stress hormones in animals by stroking them on the back 40 times a minute which is the same frequency we use in petting them. (51)

Recall the example cited above of how equestrian therapists using these techniques have been able to skillfully rehabilitate rescue horses and how they in turn successfully use these very animals to help heal autism and many other diseases as well. (91)

A TRUSTING HORMONE

Research is showing that oxytocin is far more than a hormone of labor and lactation. It can also shut down the body's most powerful defense system, that of "fight or flight". Special cerebral scans demonstrate that raising oxytocin levels makes people more trusting and trustworthy and quiets brain centers. This hormone has undoubtedly helped man during the long, stressful Ice Age during which the triumph of trust over paranoia helped both humans and animals come together in domesticated partnerships. These partnerships enabled and engendered the development of harmonious civilized life, and still enable it today. (51)

A FRIENDSHIP HORMONE

Oxytocin is a powerful means of drawing humans together and making us feel better in one another's company. Best friendships with both humans and animals were born in a vast natural landscape and on man's cultivations that followed. In such a setting we have been steeped in oxytocin for the past 10,000 years. (51)

MADE FOR EACH OTHER

Olmert notes that keeping animals and their submitting to our care has created a powerful feedback system that changed our hearts and minds. The physiological reality of why animals can love us and we can love them seems to have been identified in this marvelous hormone and gives great credence to the concept that love is good for everyone it touches. The animals painted along with humans on rock walls of prehistoric caves lends strong support to the sense that we really were made for each other. (51)

WE HAVE CONFIRMATION

The quiet trust that is so evident in a weaned child resting in its mother's lap may be a lingering effect of oxytocin that was produced in both by breast feeding.(92)

WHAT A LIST OF BENEFITS !

In summary, as more and more of our world becomes paved and polluted, our uncontrollable desire is to keep pets as well as to yearn for the out-of-doors. Keeping animals and interacting with the out-of-doors and God's creatures fills us with joy. Animals are wonderful and powerful antidotes to the poison of modern day stress and disease. Gardens and animals help heal us and can help children with autism immensely. Oxytocin and its generation from animal contacts is a great gift from God. It helps children with ASDs to recover their health and it promotes their social interaction. In truth, it engenders sociability in all of us. Oxytocin bolsters our immune systems and makes us good caregivers, not only of animals, but of each other as well.(51)

IT'S NATURAL LAW

We are a hungry nation, and one of the least recognized, yet most powerful, hungers is not one for food but for one that resides deep in our hearts. This is the powerful hunger to somehow be back home on the land and to live unhurried and secure.(51) We ourselves may not have been raised in such a setting but, in another sense, we all have come from there, even though a thousand years may have slipped away since. Or, perhaps, we really were there "relatively" recently, for when our country was founded, 95% of the population lived outside of cities on farms (93). Thus, coming back to living on the land could certainly be considered a real "coming home."

Truly, the small family garden farm is the natural habitat of the family. It is its cradle and its cure.

Chapter Six

The Canary Children

The Problem

EVERYONE IS DIFFERENT INSIDE

In Chapter One, we discussed the ability the human body has to detoxify and excrete noxious substances, such as mercury and lead, and emphasized that the ability of individuals to accomplish this varies widely. So, depending on a particular person's level of noxious substances (toxins or poisons) and the ability to excrete them, the person may experience no problems at all, minor problems, or even severe health consequences. I am convinced that children with autism are in poor health because the level of noxious substances they harbor far exceeds their capability to detoxify and remove. This situation is frequently complicated by the fact that most adults, like my wife Jill, whose health was suddenly affected by this type of malady, are completely unaware of what is causing the problem. Furthermore, they have no idea of what to do in order to regain and safeguard their health. In the same manner, the parents of children with autism typically do not understand the likely causes of autism or what they can do to remedy the problem.

CANARIES --THE FIRST TO SUFFER

The fact that some people are much more susceptible to noxious substances than others can be illustrated by an analogous situation that routinely occurred in the past, and still occasionally occurs in today's underground mines. A major dangerous condition developed in mines, particularly after a fire or an underground explosion. The resulting level of poisonous gases would climb to levels sufficient to kill miners who were exposed to them for more than a short time. However, the miners were unable to sense the presence of these toxic agents sufficiently early to escape. Canaries were found to be very sensitive to poisonous gases. They quickly suffered adverse effects or died when exposed to them. Therefore, the practice of taking a caged canary into the mine and observing it closely was adopted. Distress or death of the canary provided a signal for the miners to exit immediately or suffer the same fate.

A NEAR- PERFECT ANALOGY

Children with autism can be likened to the canaries taken into the mines. But, they are infinitely more precious and by no means expendable. Because these little ones are more sensitive to noxious substances, they become ill when exposed to levels that most individuals can tolerate. Their immune systems also become out-of-balance (a condition known as dysregulation). This imbalance often leads to many conditions, including rashes, allergies, and infections. In this chapter, we will explore the close relationship between the immune system and the liver. We also discuss the stress that results when the liver is overburdened beyond its ability to do its job. We will call attention to the extra work thrust on the immune system and the liver when stressors overwhelm them and cause their functions to decline.

WHERE IS THE EXIT DOOR?

Please note that our affected children resemble canaries, even to their confinement in cages. Unlike canaries in mines, however, these precious little ones are by no means expendable indicators of a dangerous atmosphere.

You and I have the ability to open the cage door, pictured on the front cover of this book. However, releasing a distressed canary *inside* the mine would not save it. Therefore, we doorkeepers, just as those miners, must have the good sense to exit our own toxic environment quickly and take our little canaries with us if they are to be rescued and freed to fly away. The toxic environment of which we speak is the polluted world around us, as described in the *Dark Skies and Dirty Water* chapter. It also includes the conditions within our bodies of a dysbiotic, leaky intestine, a clogged liver filter, and the consequent dysregulated immunity.

WHAT IS THE IMMUNE SYSTEM?

The immune system is a collection of tissue that serves as the armed forces of the body. Its basic orders are to identify and eliminate foreign and harmful substances and microorganisms that have invaded the body. Unlike the heart or the stomach, the immune system doesn't have a single anatomic location. It is distributed throughout the body because, in order to fulfill its function, it must be at all places at all times. It contains specialized cells that produce antibodies or ingest foreign invaders in a perpetual "search and destroy" mission. Some of the white blood cells assigned to this function circulate in the blood stream. These circulating white blood cells are always on a surveillance mission in order to handle a problem where and when it begins. Other white cells are "stay at homes." These are stationed in the reticuloendothelial (R-E) organs of the body, including the liver, spleen, bone marrow, thymus gland, and the lymphatic system. This lymphatic system is widely distributed throughout the body. It includes the gut-associated lymphoid tissue (G.A.L.T.) and the mucosa associated lymphatic system (M.A.L.T.) in our intestines. Remarkably, the majority of our immune system resides in our intestinal tract. (94)

THE LIVER—CENTRAL TO AUTISM

The liver protects the immune system from overload because it serves as the body's great filter. (95) It also processes fats, carbohydrates, and proteins as well as hormones. It stores vitamins, participates in digestion, and detoxifies medicines and harmful chemicals.(96) If we wish to effectively combat autism, we must acknowledge two realities. The first reality is that the liver is usually laboring in a state of overload much greater than most people can imagine. The second reality is that the central role of the liver in the lives of children with autism, and really in all our lives, is poorly recognized and poorly understood, even by most professionals who undertake the treatment of this disorder. We need to begin attending to these realities.

WHO WILL BE NEXT ?

Our first step should be to appreciate that we are all, in a sense, potentially "autistic". As our world becomes increasingly uninhabitable, nature has been busy looking for adult equivalents of autism with which to warn us. One of those signals is the siren sound of sterility in man and beast alike. Another is Alzheimer's disease. A third is schizophrenia.

WORDS OF WISDOM

Dr. Sandra Cabot, the experienced and internationally recognized physician from Australia who contributed the Forward to this book, also wrote the following very helpful words.

> "In life, real solutions are generally simple…and they are logical and practical.
>
> "They must also be easy to follow, otherwise they will fall by the wayside and be thrown into the 'too hard' basket. I must admit it took me more than twenty years of medical practice before the solution dawned on me! The liver, the supreme organ of metabolism, had to be the missing key. It seems so simple and so obvious and yet so incredible; why hadn't someone thought of this before?" (97)

A STRONG RECOMMENDATION

Dr. Cabot has "seen the light" and she fights the battle to focus that light on the liver. In fact, her effective regimen of a special diet, presented in the books she has written, and potent non-prescription liver-supporting supplements are "just what the doctor ordered" for all of us. Her regimen especially fits children with autism, ADHD, and their mothers. Parents of these children would be wise to have them follow the same diet and supplement plan that she herself uses. Parents-to-be, who wish to avoid the problem of autism and ADHD in their children should also use this regimen. Dr. Cabot's recommended measures can, and should, begin prior to conception.

DON'T LET THE KNOWLEDGE GO TO WASTE

Dr. Cabot has written several books on how to care for the liver and preserve its function, along with books that discuss other very important medical topics, such as obesity and infertility. Her unique approach has proven so effective that it occupies an important place in the management of autism we are recommending here. All the principles and recipes that she espouses are safe to apply to children. (98,99) Dr. Cabot has kindly composed a synopsis of her view of autism in the Introduction to this book. The reader is well advised to look deeply into the library of medical topics authored by this experienced clinician. Her books are well written and very easy to understand. Many millions of people from all over the world have benefited from her knowledge and approach.

ALL EYES ON THE LIVER

At the end of Chapter One, we made reference to the effect of genetically transmitted impairments in detoxification pathways (e.g. the folic acid- and vitamin B-12-dependent methylation pathway Dr. Cave mentioned in her Introduction to this book) and to effects of these impairments on the accumulation of poisons. In this chapter, we emphasize that the liver is where the majority of these processes occur. This organ is, thus, a critical determinant of how well our body rids itself of noxious or harmful agents accumulating from within the body or from the environment. A critical factor in disarming and eliminating these poisons is the condition of the liver. It is the Grand Central Station in this process. The ancients said: "All roads lead to Rome." the empire we call our body, all detoxification pathways lead to the liver.

A VERY IMPORTANT TRUTH REVEALED

No matter what kind of contaminants enter the body, and no matter how they enter, whether through the water, the air, the skin, through food, or medicine (in both prescriptions and over-the-counter products), they pass into the bloodstream and end up in the body's filter: the liver. The liver traps these poisons, inactivates them, and prepares them for elimination from the body. The liver is the gateway to the rest of the body. However, in this chemical age its detoxification systems are easily overloaded.(100)

THE CUMULATIVE LOAD DOES IT

In a recent presentation, Dr. William Shaw of Great Plains Laboratory ascribed the low autism rate in Cuba to the tightly controlled and infrequent use of acetaminophen (also called paracetamol) in that country.(86) He connected acetaminophen use to liver damage and ascribed the biochemical pathways of this damage to the development of autism. This should not be interpreted to mean that the use of this pain killer and agent, used widely to control fever, is the only cause of autism. Shaw also acknowledges the interplay of genetic factors in the problem. To illustrate how autism likely has many causes, imagine the body's detoxification machinery --especially the liver-- as a light truck overloaded with bricks. The truck will break down whether or not all the bricks are identical. In fact, the addition of a large chunk of concrete may be the immediate cause that puts the truck out of commission.

UNLOAD BEFORE THE TIRES GO FLAT

Many experts dealing with autism agree that it is unlikely to have a single cause. Rather, just like the overloaded truck, it develops after the liver and the immune system succumb to overload. In one sense, the specific overloading factors don't really matter. The liver is broken and needs to be fixed. In another sense, identifying causes is important so they then can be avoided or eliminated.

THE FILTER CONCEPT

The liver's entrapment or filtering step in this process is similar to what occurs in the lymphatic system. Our many lymph nodes (also called lymph glands) are interconnected by specialized channels filled with lymph fluid. Lymph nodes perform a filtering function to stop cancer cells or infections from spreading throughout the body. (101) For example, if an infection were to develop in our hand, its spread into the body can be seen by the inflammation of the lymph channels that appear as red streaks moving up the arm.

A REAL PROCESSING PLANT

Here the similarity between the lymph nodes and the liver ends. While both the lymph nodes and the liver function as filters, only the liver entraps the material, then processes and readies it for elimination. This "garbage" is bagged and prepared for trucking to the dump. Both the bagging process and the outward movement (called excretion) occur in the liver. One can begin to understand the liver's great importance by considering that, in addition to the critical nature of its filtering process, the liver also has about 500 other known functions.(96)

THE LIVER HAS ITS LIMITS

The liver also contains its own blood and lymphatic, fluid-filled channels, called sinusoids. Within these spaces specially modified white blood cells, called Kupffer cells, engulf and ingest dead cells, cancer cells, yeasts, viruses, bacteria, parasites, artificial chemicals, incompletely digested proteins, and dangerous foreign particles. Once ingested, the dangerous cells are chewed up inside the Kupffer cells and put to rest. However, if these PacMan-like cells are worked too hard for too long, they may become so overburdened with toxins that the liver's task of keeping the bloodstream clean can no longer be fully achieved. In such cases many different symptoms of poor health may occur, such as allergies, headaches, and chronic fatigue. This is the body's equivalent of what happens in a neighborhood during a garbage collection strike when deteriorating waste collects everywhere.(98,102,103)

A WORD ABOUT OUR BOWELS

At this point I should address a common misconception with regard to the role of the bowels. The bowels are primarily a channel of elimination. Their prime role is not to cleanse, filter, or remove toxic wastes from the bloodstream, (102) but the health of our liver, lymphatic system, and immune system are greatly affected by the state of our intestines. (96)

THE BREAKDOWN DESCRIBED

The liver is the hardest working organ in the body, especially in our increasingly toxic environment. (97,104) It must cope with every chemical and poison we encounter, including drugs, both prescription and over-the-counter, the damaged fats present in fried and processed foods, the excess refined carbohydrates in sodas, cookies, or other dessert-type foods, as well as with too many alcoholic drinks (Appendix C). If persons expose themselves to an excess amount of these types of chemicals and poisons, the overload can cause a breakdown in the liver's ability to do its job and one of its most basic jobs, which is to metabolize fat.

SYSTEM OVERLOAD, SYSTEM REPAIR

When the liver can no longer effectively metabolize fat, the excess fat accumulates and is distributed or stored between liver cells, causing the condition of a "fatty liver." Actually, storage is a convenient but not an accurate term. This burgeoning mass of stored fat isn't by any means inactive or asleep. In fact, its presence provokes an inflammatory reaction wherever it is deposited. When this storage occurs in the liver, it begins to hamper that organ's capacity to detoxify the blood. A vicious cycle results. The liver's inability to keep up with all its tasks creates a huge accumulation of fat that, in turn, causes the failing liver to weaken further. Unfortunately, it is not uncommon to find a fatty liver in adolescents who consume a diet high in processed and fast foods. (105) In contrast, juicing and the ingestion of raw foods improves the liver's ability to burn fats. A diet that cleanses the liver can generally rejuvenate those in poor health, even poor health from unknown causes. (106)

A MATTER OF DEGREES

Fatty liver is known in medical circles as "non-alcoholic fatty liver disease," and this is often abbreviated to NAFLD. The term includes the condition of "simple fatty liver" but also incorporates a more severe condition abbreviated as NASH. The difference between a simple fatty liver and NASH is the degree of inflammation present. As inflammation increases, scarring develops throughout the liver, eventually resulting in cirrhosis. (107) This material is relevant to adult women who wish to make their livers healthy in order to bear healthy children.

A FILTER THAT CLEANS ITSELF

You may think that this is an over simplification. It is not. Because the liver is the body's great filter, it must be in tip top shape to strain out all the contaminants that reach it through the body's many entrances. A cleansing and maintenance process, to be addressed later, is a big part of the solution.

PROTECT IT, CARE FOR IT, LOVE IT

I believe that many physicians in the United States do not appreciate the liver as the most strategic organ in the body. Thus, this very important organ does not receive the consideration it deserves. Our liver protects our body "24/7" from untold harmful agents, and we are well-advised to keep it working efficiently.(98)

THEY CAN TAKE ONLY SO MUCH

In today's modern environment, a child's body, and really most adult bodies, labor under a handicap. All the contaminants that have entered the body from the outside and have filled up or congested the body's liver and packed it full of unnatural substances are oftentimes chemicals new to the body. It is a difficult task for the liver to process these foreign and oftentimes very potent substances. As a consequence, they remain trapped in the liver for years, adding to the congestion and further blocking its filtering function. (34,102) This results in toxins slipping past the liver and circulating in the blood from which they are deposited in cells throughout the body. As they accumulate in the brain and in other organs, they produce all kinds of problems, including inflammation, illnesses, and --plausibly-- autism.

Reader, please note how the brain can be exposed to harmful environmental agents that the liver has failed to remove. Due to their high fat composition, the brain, pituitary, thyroid, adrenals, testes, and ovaries are predisposed to this deposition.

LONG AWAITED CONFIRMATION

Our government recognized the need to study a possible causal link between autism and single or combined genetic, biologic, and environmental factors in a report from a 2011 workshop on the increasing autism rate in the US.(108) More important yet, a report by Stanford University researchers gives substantial support to the role of the environment in causing autism. In a study involving twins in which at least one of the pair had autism, the findings showed that genes accounted for 38% of autism risk in the children they studied, with environmental factors explaining the remaining 62%.

In an interview, two of the investigators mentioned that their work pointed to environmental risk factors causing something to happen in early life perhaps even during pregnancy, and one of these scientists recommended that events during pregnancy should be a focus for future research into the origins of autism. (109) I contend that how both the mother's and the baby's liver handle these environmental toxins is the key issue. It is precisely here that our attention must be directed.

THEY END UP IN THE BRAIN

Most toxic chemicals are non-polar or fat-soluble. This means that they don't mix well with water. Instead, they form bubbles or films when added to water. An example of this would be the multicolored film that forms when a small amount of motor oil or gasoline falls on a puddle of water. When non-polar toxic chemicals enter the body, the liver is less able to deactivate them and make them soluble in water. Therefore, they can't be excreted. If they were water soluble, they could be excreted as they normally are via aqueous fluids, such as urine, bile, and sweat. But, because of their insolubility, they spill into the blood stream. Once in the blood stream, these toxins seek out organs with a high fat content where they are deposited. The fact that the brain composition is mostly lipid (the medical term for fat) and the endocrine organs mentioned above are high in lipid content makes these preferred organs where these toxins lodge. In other words, because these toxins are drawn to the brain like a magnet, the brain is more vulnerable to damage from these toxins than other organs in the body. This is especially true of the developing nervous systems of babies that, by virtue of their immaturity, are exquisitely sensitive to environmental chemicals.

WHEN IT'S FULL, IT'S FULL

Thus, toxins build up in the bloodstream as the liver's filter falters. They are then carried deeper into the body via the blood where they must be dealt with by the immune system. This system becomes severely stressed when the liver loses its barrier function and becomes incapable of handling increasing amounts of environmental contamination. Although the immune system protects our bodies from many dangers, it is the liver which protects the immune system from overload --unless the liver is itself overloaded.(97) And in today's world, the liver frequently is overloaded. Appendix C lists some of the many ways in which our liver can be overwhelmed.

GET TO THE ROOT OF THE PROBLEM

The immune system's suspected role in the causation of autism likely relates to the fact that, when it becomes overloaded, it also becomes irritated. In this hyperstimulated state it begins to produce excessive inflammatory chemicals and sometimes autoantibodies that are directed against our own tissue. Symptoms of immune overload include allergies, inflammatory diseases, swollen glands, recurrent infections, chronic fatigue, and autoimmune disease such as lupus, rheumatoid arthritis, or Hashimoto's thyroiditis. Rather than treating all these problems with steroids, such as cortisone or prednisone, the simplest and most efficient way to take the load off the immune system is by improving liver function. (102) Problems that are caused by an imbalance in the immune system will always, and often dramatically, improve with a diet that cleanses and improves the function of the liver. (97)

LIVER FILTER EXAMPLE # 1

A recent event in the food industry exemplifies how the liver is involved in the trapping of dangerous substances. Broiler chickens were being treated with 3-Nitro (Roxarsone) to prevent their developing intestinal tract infections. This agent contained organic arsenic that was thought to be safe in this application. However, a study by the FDA revealed that the arsenic in 3-Nitro transformed in the chicken's body into inorganic arsenic which is a known carcinogen (a chemical capable of causing cancer) for both animals and humans. Higher levels of inorganic arsenic were found in the livers of treated chickens than in untreated chickens. This finding prompted the drug's manufacturer to voluntarily suspend its sale.(110)

LIVER FILTER EXAMPLE # 2

Similarly, the State of Michigan Department of Natural Resources warns hunters not to eat the livers of game or wild fowl taken from areas watered by the Tittabawassee River downstream from Midland, MI, the location of a large chemical plant and other industrial operations, due to the presence of the poisonous chemical by-product, dioxin, concentrating in their livers.(111)

LIVER FILTER EXAMPLE # 3

An another example involves human beings. Acetaminophen -- the number one selling over-the-counter health product in the country-- crosses the placenta and is detectable in neonatal serum after birth. The unborn child's liver is especially prone to being damaged by this drug because the capacity to metabolize it doesn't begin until 18 weeks gestation. Thereafter only some of the pathways are operative in the fetus and these function at a rate that is approximately ten times slower than that in the adult liver. (86)

LIVER FILTER EXAMPLE # 4

The Food and Drug Administration (FDA) Total Diet Study

found that beef and calf liver contained 49 different pesticide residues. This was reported in a book by David Steinman entitled *Diet for a Poisoned Planet* (112) This finding is over 25 years old. One can only speculate how this contamination has worsened in the interval since then.(112) A more recent (2006) edition of this respected book continues to document a high number of unnatural contaminants in food. This is especially true of butter tested by the FDA and found to have the highest pesticide content of any dairy food.

BORN TOXIC

I will now use data already presented to provide tangible evidence that the liver as a filter is truly being overburdened. Alarmingly, this condition is already present at birth. In 2001, the Environmental Working Group found 287 chemicals in newborn umbilical cord blood of American children. Over two thirds of chemicals that they identified in umbilical cord blood are known to be toxic to the brain and nervous system. (52) The presence of these chemicals in the blood of babies is evidence of the inability of their developing livers to remove them. For the first time in the history of the world, every human being is subjected to contact with dangerous chemicals from the moment of conception until death. These chemicals are now stored in the bodies of the vast majority of human beings, regardless of age. These toxins remain in the liver and body fat of adults for years. (102,108,113) In fact, the observation that nearly 200 of these toxins have been banned from the market for years (54) suggests that the mothers may have been harboring them also and then passed them on to their babies while they were still in the womb. Many of the chemicals that we are exposed to these days, whether they are in food, medications, or in the environment as pesticides, are newly created molecules that may take up to 40 years for the body to break down.(108) As the environment becomes ever more polluted, so do our bodies.(114) At the end of this discussion we will propose a program of how mothers can reverse this damage in their children's livers --and in their own as well-- and literally nurse them back to health.

THE BEGINNING OF THE END OF AUTISM

Because of this tragic situation, this book proposes testing the liver function of a group of newborns to investigate the possibility that the livers of those babies who later develop autism are more compromised in function at birth than the livers of babies who develop normally. Unfortunately, we believe this is quite likely to be the case, the reason being that the characteristically increased sensitivity of children with autism to environmental toxins places them at extreme risk of additional loss of liver function. Such loss of function could follow exposure to any agent imposing a toxic or an immunologic burden, such as infections or immunizations, on their frail livers. How the data from this study will be used is described later in this chapter.

SCREEN TEST FIRST

In addition, I propose that all newborns be screened for their ability to handle a potential vaccination load. Based on my testing of children with autism, I feel certain that one, two, or at most three tests could be performed to screen the newborns to ascertain the condition of the newborn's liver, detoxification mechanisms, and the baby's ability to deal with such insults as the immense immunologic challenge from multiple vaccinations given simultaneously. However, as noted above, a study will have to be done on a group of newborns before it can be determined which tests would be the best. It is just a matter of having professionals in this field of expertise develop an ethical study plan that is in line with current government recommendations involving immunizations.

Clearly, the children who develop autism will test differently than those who do not, for their bodies are weaker and more frail. So it is just a matter of determining what medical test or tests, using a blood or urine sample, will best indicate the newborn's capability to tolerate the recommended vaccination burden. In light of the information presented above, such testing of newborns might well include an assessment of the liver. Appendix D lists some candidate screening tests for newborns. It also includes two very important cautions about how these suggestions are to be used. As mentioned elsewhere in this book, the ultimate decision regarding the selection of screening tests for newborns belongs in the hands of experts.

A WEAK CHILD GETS SPECIAL TREATMENT

Checking all newborns is essential because at this age the diagnosis of autism is difficult to make and is usually deferred until the child is older. By that time, many immunizations might have already been given according to the recommended schedule. In that case, the opportunity to defer or relax the schedule of administration to prevent potential adverse effects caused by their routine administration will have been lost. This recommendation for newborn testing finds relevance in that it proposes a plan to prevent the development of autism in the face of its tragically high current incidence and the extreme difficulty encountered in trying to reverse vaccine-related damage in affected children.

SOME WEAK, SOME STRONG

Fortunately, there is great hope for the future. It is now a well-proven fact that we all respond to environmental agents and drugs differently due both to our genetic make up and to how well each of our organs is working. Hopefully, the knowledge of our biochemical uniqueness --and the ability to detect it based on the assessment of the function of the individual's liver-- will bring a quick end to the "one size fits all" approach in childhood vaccinations. The era of the analysis of each individual's genetic makeup is fast upon us. Scientific articles are beginning to appear that predict the effectiveness or intolerance of some treatment based on an individual's gene makeup.

EPIGENETICS

However, even more important than knowing our genetic makeup is the scientifically proven finding that the expression of our genes is dependent on our nutrition. Dr. Cabot alluded to this important fact in her Forward. This phenomenon is called Epigenetics (115,116) Specific nutrients are required to turn our genes on and off, thus regulating their activities. Without the correct nutrition, our genes and the chromosomes on which they reside would not be able to influence our lives any more than a printed circuit in an electronic device can cause it to function when that device is disconnected from any power source. Our liver manufactures, stores, and/or orchestrates the activities of many, if not all, of these key gene-regulating nutrients as another of its numerous functions.

LIKE MOTHER, LIKE CHILD

Dr. Cabot notes that about one third of all the patients she sees have at least some degree of liver dysfunction, that is, loss of function. Her experience is mirrored by that of a pathologist with whom I spoke who noted the presence of a vast amount of advanced liver disease of unknown cause. As liver problems are common (105,117), it isn't surprising that pregnant mothers whose livers aren't working properly can pass toxins of all sorts to the babies inside of them through the placenta.

MOTHERLY CARE

Obviously, a mother must take care of her body during

pregnancy and even before, for that matter. Most mothers do a great job of this and that's probably why so many fewer babies have autism at present. The point is made that many reasons exist that can cause a child to develop autism, as discussed throughout this book. However, if a mother is not careful in caring for herself, this can result in autism in her child. All mothers need to understand that caring for their own health is so important in these times because of all the unnatural contaminants coming into their bodies through the food, the environment, and even the medicines they may take in excess amounts.

A REVEALING EXAMPLE

Below is an example of how a mother who has not cared for herself can cause her liver to become overburdened, and how this can harm her baby.

MOTHER, TAKE CARE OF YOUR LIVER

The mother's liver must work hard to break down female hormones which reach high levels during pregnancy. In addition, today we are immersed in environmental chemicals such as pesticides and plastics, some of which have estrogenic activity. The added burden imposed by these foreign estrogens may be sufficient to swamp the hormonal breakdown pathways in the mother's liver if she has not taken good care of herself, for example, by drinking large amounts of diet soda to keep from gaining weight. This happens because the aspartame used by most brands as a sweetener is known to be toxic to the liver. Also, if the mother has had to take an excess amount of medicines, she exposes herself to liver damage from the heavy use of acetaminophen present in over-the-counter and prescription pain and headache medicine, and from other drugs.

IN THESE TIMES ESPECIALLY

All mothers must be aware of the danger to the child living inside of them and overcome the natural tendencies to eat poorly which results in having to take excess medication during pregnancy. In these times, many of the foods, drinks, and medicines are so unnatural that they act to congest the liver, as this discussion attempts to make clear. However, if yielding to natural tendencies and the inordinate use of unnatural substances prevail, then this huge workload of metabolizing estrogens and chemicals behaving as estrogens is thrust on a mother's liver that is quite likely already damaged.

AND TO MAKE MATTERS WORSE

Add to this the nutritional deficiencies afflicting a mother who does not take care of herself that further cripples the liver's ability to function. This sets the stage for this mother to pass an excess amount of these toxins to the baby in her uterus through the placenta and, after birth, to the baby through the breast milk.

HOW VACCINATIONS MAY CAUSE AUTISM

In this example, if the baby's liver is overburdened with toxins coming from a mother who has not taken good care of herself, the baby's liver is far too underdeveloped and already too overworked to handle them. It will mean the accumulation of additional harmful substances entering the baby's body. Due to the baby's frail and faltering liver, these toxins then spill over into the baby's own bloodstream. Once the additional harmful substances are in the baby's bloodstream, they will pass deeply into the body to his or her other underdeveloped organs which are also extremely vulnerable to damage. The liver's job is to protect the immune system from damage, but the baby's liver is in a weakened state because of its "inherited" toxic load and is, in addition, low in essential nutrients.

Therefore, it will be impossible in situations such as these for the baby's liver and immune system to function properly. For example, vaccination ingredients might get distributed throughout the baby's body instead of being correctly processed in the liver and in other parts of the immune system. The infant's body will look upon this foreign material injected into it as one more substance to worsen its overload, risking damage to the liver itself and to every organ to which it is carried by the bloodstream, including the brain. Under the circumstances outlined here, the baby sees the vaccination as another toxic substance. Therefore, his or her organs react to and are at risk of being harmed by the vaccination ingredients just as they would be by any toxin. The harm of which we speak may be, in other terms, autism.

The Solution

HOW WE MAY BE ABLE TO PREVENT AUTISM

Suppose, however, we could predict in advance, on the basis of the limited test panel advocated above, the capacity of the baby's liver to handle the cumulative load placed upon it by an untimely and aggressive vaccination schedule. Then, it would be possible to determine which children are not likely to be able to handle or process the standard regimen of shots. In this event, an adjustment in the vaccination schedule could be made by creating a program of immunizations that the liver might reasonably be expected to handle. This approach has some precedent. The CDC provides recommendations for amending the vaccination schedule in children with immune deficiency diseases, many of which are of genetic origin (118) The approach I present here differs from that of the CDC because I recommend the deciding factor be based on the liver's metabolic and biochemical capacity to withstand multiple, simultaneous immunizations given at an early age.

Perhaps fewer vaccinations would be given at one time, or the vaccination schedule could be delayed until the liver test results showed some improvement. Would we then see fewer cases of autism developing? In my opinion, we would in a great way. Such a plan involving modification of how vaccines would be administered has been proposed by other writers. For example, in her book *Gut and Psychology Syndrome* Natasha Campbell McBride, M.D. recommends a parental health history questionnaire be completed before an infant is vaccinated and that this measure be accompanied by a comprehensive stool and urine analysis to assess any risk of gut dysbiosis in the baby, as well as a test to assess the infant's immune status.(119) Along the same lines, one of the pediatricians whom I mentioned in Chapter Two recommends that the prospective mother undergo a proprietary cleanse before becoming pregnant.

PRESENT DANGER SET

It is helpful to note that the medical and pharmaceutical professions have adjusted medical injections for years based on the capacity of a sick person to tolerate them. For example, they might decrease the amount and frequency of an antibiotic that could further harm the kidney in an individual with compromised kidney function. Measures like these seem to work quite well in preventing further damage to a compromised organ. Also, today it is standard practice to first make sure that a patient's liver function is normal with laboratory tests before administering a prescription medication which has the potential to damage the liver. Such screening is unlikely to occur, however, with over-the counter products. Based on the above evidence, it would seem to make great sense to test newborns' liver function and perhaps also gain some indication of their toxic load before introducing further substances into their systems, agents that might have the effect of seriously affecting their health and perhaps even cause them to develop autism. As noted above, such a recommendation is not without precedent. Recall the CDC recommends omitting some --or even all-- immunizations in some rare diseases of deficient immune function. (118) The tenet of this book is that immune dysfunction is common in infants and children and that this disorder is secondary to, that is, caused by a malfunctioning liver.

KNOWLEDGE IS USELESS IF NOT USED

In 2001 a study based on a telephone survey disclosed that nearly one-quarter of all parents felt that their children were receiving more vaccinations than were good for them. (120) The following year, 2002, the prestigious Institute of Medicine (IOM), the medical branch of the National Academy of Sciences, issued a report on the deleterious effect that multiple immunizations may have on the immune system of young children. Because there were no available studies to review, the IOM Committee members stated that they were unable to ascertain the risk of immune or nervous system damage, or death itself, when multiple vaccinations are administered to a susceptible or frail child. In addition to encouraging more research on the development of the human infant's immune system, the Committee, allowing for the vulnerability of some newborns to multiple immunizations, recommended a more flexible schedule be developed to decrease the number of vaccines administered at one time. (121)

SIDESTEPPING THE ISSUE

In August, 2011, a more recent IOM review found vaccine complications were rare and usually reversible. However, the review did not address the health effects of multiple vaccinations given together.(122) Thus, this report completely sidestepped the issue of the vaccination cumulative load discussed in this chapter and in Chapter 2 of this book. This cumulative load concept seems to be of critical importance in the development of autism.

IT'S TIME TO FOLLOW THROUGH

A decade has passed since the 2002 IOM report. In that interval, the incidence of autism has skyrocketed, environmental pollution has intensified daily, the number of recommended immunizations has increased, and the American diet continues to deteriorate with the main meal of the day often being take-out food. Certainly, the number of frail newborns with damaged livers and weak immune systems also must be growing. The recommendation of the IOM in 2002 for development of a more flexible approach to when and how many vaccinations are given is more relevant now than ever.

TAKE OFF THE BLINDERS

I realize that many physicians and health authorities believe that no connection exists between immunizations and autism. But the experience of parents who have witnessed the scourge of autism develop in their children immediately following a vaccination, especially in the time just before two years of age, argues for a connection with equal certainty and a good measure of heartache. There are also many physicians who are very concerned about the "safety" of vaccinations and, like the physicians referred to earlier, have developed what they feel is a "safe" way to vaccinate.

THE ANSWER

I will now propose an approach, one that should be acceptable to all, and one that addresses both the possible cause and a means of prevention of autism. The novelty of our proposal lies in the emphasis it places on healthy liver function, in addition to other parameters, both in mother and child, beginning before conception and continuing throughout nursing. In one important application, this method would give a green light to infant vaccinations after two determinations have been made:

> I. The identification of several tests that, by retrospective analysis, are able to predict which individual is likely to suffer an adverse reaction (including autism) following vaccinations.
>
> II. The little baby lying before us does not have an abnormality in any of those tests.

The approach that I am advocating does not argue against vaccinating our children but urges us to take into account the fact that we are all biochemically unique and, thus, different. It only stands to reason that such differences must be considered *before* the administration of vaccinations. Persons from many different walks of life with whom we have discussed this proposal have, without exception, thought it to be reasonable and worthwhile.

THE FACT OF THE MATTER

I am firmly convinced that the condition of each individual's organ system, especially the liver, determines a person's ability to tolerate a certain number of vaccinations and when they can be given. If that number or time is not respected, then for some children the shots cease to be medicine and instead become poison. No longer a benefit, they may cause the children to suffer serious and perhaps irreversible damage. Either we confer immunity or cause injury.

PLACE THE CHILDREN FIRST

Hopefully, professionals in this field of expertise will accept and act on this proposal to test all newborns in the manner described above. I submit that all those who are responsible for the lives and well-being of defenseless children are accountable to the Author of Life, and are duty-bound to cooperate with such a testing program and follow the recommendation stemming from it. Let not convenience, nor profiteering, nor bad science, nor closed-mindedness, nor time-urgency-driven medical care that runs more by rote than by reason stand in the path of doing what, in the view of this book, is best for our children.

HOW TO HEAL A BABY'S LIVER

All are very aware of how cautious physicians are in prescribing medications to lactating mothers because of the possibility of exposing the nursing infant to whatever substance the mother consumes. In my practice, a nursing infant developed a rash whenever the mother ate peanut butter. Conversely, it is very plausible that by following the principles of *The Liver Cleansing Diet* and using one of the liver-restoring supplements Dr. Cabot recommends a mother could through her breast milk impart healing to her baby's liver, shown to be weak by testing. Dr. Cabot emphasizes that the nursing mother's diet also be rich in vitamin C, selenium, and other antioxidants. Then future testing will hopefully show that the state of this baby's liver has improved to the point where some immunizations may be administered, perhaps those designed to prevent the diseases that used to be commonplace and that made children very ill. The specific prioritization of immunizations is left to those who are well-versed in the prevention of the contagious diseases of childhood.

GET IN SHAPE, MOM

Finally, mothers with liver dysfunction, uncovered by similar testing and desiring to prevent autism from developing in their child, might reasonably defer becoming pregnant until nutritional remediation with *The Liver Cleansing Diet* and repeat testing confirm that the future mother's liver is again healthy.

LIVER HEALTH THE KEY

All this being true, the first step on the road to recovery, for both children and adults, is to put the liver back in shape. In other words, clean out the filter and provide what it needs to work in a perfect way. Then the liver can do its job and keep contaminants from circulating in the blood and ending up in brain cells and elsewhere in the body. If the liver is healthy enough to filter out all the contaminants, they will exit the body by normal means. We should all be aware that the liver's function as a filter requires some regular maintenance, as any filter would, especially in today's very toxic environment. The liver can become plugged up and need cleansing on a regular basis. It is like the oil filter on your car engine. One big difference is that it is a lot easier to change the oil filter in your car than it is to change your liver. (95,102) So we had better take good care of our original equipment!

Having worked in molecular biology early in my career, I certainly appreciate the importance of the genes. The medical journals and the internet are teeming with reports of how SNPs, or little defects in our DNA, can predispose us to this or that disease. However, the big picture which reveals that the diseases which kill most of us result from our inability to control the quantity of food we consume, worsened by its poor nutritional quality and toxicity. And the organ that takes the first hit in all this, the hypocenter, the ground zero, is our great filter, the liver. "Love your liver and live," Dr. Cabot urges. (123) We haven't heeded her admonition. Our devitalized, chemical, junk-in-junk-out daily fare just isn't fair to our livers. Its manufacturer's warranty has run out. And the time left for us in which to begin mindful eating is close behind. As noted in Chapter Five, infertility is rampant in both animals and humans. Our future, indeed the very survival of the human race, is teetering precariously on the tip of our forks. Let this dictum dominate every domain and direct our decisions at dinner.

CARE FOR YOUR LIVER

True, a filter has to be renewed and is sometimes damaged and needs to be replaced, at least part of it. But the best way to care for it is to never let it get so impaired that it cannot be renewed and put back into tip top shape. Our Creator has provided a way to do this.

KEEP THE FILTER CLEAN

Just as we would never think of replacing the oil in our car engine with anything but clean, pure, new motor oil, nor ever put water or grime into the car's gas tank, so too we should eat only fresh, pure food, free of artificial or unnatural contaminants. But today's world is not perfect and we have pollution of all sorts entering our bodies in many ways. So we have to do periodic cleansing of the filter and provide what it needs to stay in good operating condition our whole life long. This can be done and it must be the approach to the problem of contaminants that could cause autism and many other illnesses related to our toxic environment of soil, water, and air.

THE RECOMMENDED PROGRAM

In short, Dr. Cabot's program entails de-stressing the liver by consuming healthy foods, raw juices, and natural medicines from the garden that are intended to relieve the intense workload of the liver. At the same time, her program provides purifying and remedial nutrients, especially those that are known to support the liver and to restore its natural filter function. Important ingredients in this regimen are several, carefully designed formulations. It is important to note that all of Dr. Cabot's principles are safe to apply to children, and the liver supplements may be administered to them directly after the age of two or three. (98,99) Her *Liver Cleansing Diet* is the only scientific eating plan devised by a physician to improve liver function. (117) I frequently recommend Dr. Cabot's books to patients and friends and even arrange to have it sent to those whom I believe could benefit from it. I hope you will also.

LOTS OF CLEANING TO DO

A frail newborn's body was created only to tolerate mother's milk. Vaccinations certainly weren't in the original plan. The newborn liver is still being formed, and yet, as noted above, the newborn's liver often is clogged from the start. It is essential to remove the poisons from the body in order to allow new cells, including those in the brain, to develop. As it stands now, the whole body has toxic trash spread throughout its trillions of cells. If autism is to be prevented, infants need a cleanup beginning with the liver and starting early in life. First the blood will be cleansed, and then all the poisons stored in body cells. A liver-friendly regimen is the key. The whole approach consists of the diet and the kind of liver-healing substances Dr. Cabot uses in her formulations. For the very young, the plan is for the mother first to cleanse her liver and then to cleanse the baby and, as stated above, literally nurse her child back to health.

THE BODY MUST HAVE WHAT IT NEEDS TO FUNCTION

Additional aid is also needed that is also just as important to ensure the body has all the nutrients it needs to function perfectly. Many doctors who are trying hard to help children with autism recommend or prescribe many supplements. As a result, the families or parents are stressed to the limit by having to purchase them to help their children. And in almost all cases, children do benefit from these supplements. Ideally, the children and adults would not need any supplements. The reason the supplements are necessary the majority of the time is because of the lack of nutrients in the food supply.

A SAD SITUATION: NATIONAL HEALTH WORSENS

Everything begins with the soil, as explained in a Chapter 5, *Help from the Barn*. The soil in this country has been depleted of the nutrients it needs. President FDR warned us long ago that a nation that destroys its soil destroys itself. Sir Albert Howard ends his book with a similar dire admonition. (85) Our farm soil is being cared for improperly and, worse still, it is being contaminated daily with fertilizer-filler material in the form of industrial waste and unnatural chemicals. Some of these are added to the ground to help farmers do more work in less time and have greater yields. It is apparent that many in the food chain are motivated by profit and not by the quality of the food produced. The result is that the food eaten in this country is deficient in the nutrients needed by human bodies. As a result, health care costs have skyrocketed out of control and the people are suffering, our little canaries the worst.

THE RIGHT WAY, THE BEST WAY

Those who have to live in apartments with no land to keep animals and grow their own food have to do the best they can with the purchase of organic foods and supplements. However, those who live in the countryside can do what they can to keep animals, add supplements to their food, and raise their own food in fields and garden soils nurtured with natural supplements, mostly minerals from the sea. The harvested crops and animal products grown under these conditions will have all the nutrients needed by the body and, in addition, the food will be free of all contaminants. This is the ideal. This is what the goal should be and, to whatever degree a family achieves this goal, will be the degree that they will profit with good health in body and in mind.

WE HAVE PROOF

At this point, I call the reader's attention to the Price-Pottinger Nutritional Foundation. (124) The books available through this foundation, especially those written by or about families living a natural lifestyle, describe how living off the land and consuming all the nutrients that human beings need can have healthy and strong bodies. In the early part of the last century Dr. Weston A. Price proved this by studying remote peoples not yet affected by the modern world. He found that peoples who raised their own food in healthy environments far from the modern world were uniformly very healthy. The pictures of people in his book prove his case over and over again. He also addresses the reason that food decreases in nutritional value as the soil is depleted of minerals. The good news is that our human bodies can thrive and babies fed properly from birth will return to the natural health they were designed to have.

THOSE WHO LIVE IN THE CITIES

So this is the answer. Just fix the liver and all else should fall into line. For the transition period and for those who have to live in apartments in big cities and don't even have yards in which to plant gardens, I will propose an alternate regimen. This should make it possible for everyone to have a treatment plan for reversing or preventing ill health, including autism.

NO GETTING AROUND THE FACTS

Any approach to the management or prevention of autism requires recognition that the human body must have whatever it needs to work and function each day. Most people fail in this regard and their bodies suffer as a consequence. Although the illness that results is quite evident and people realize the shortcomings in the Western diet, few persons make the necessary effort to ensure their bodies have all the essential nutrients needed to maintain health. Fewer still make the necessary effort to avoid consuming toxins or poisons.

WHY SPECIAL CARE FOR CHILDREN WITH AUTISM

However, when caring for a child with autism, a parent cannot overlook the glaring defectiveness of our food supply. The parents of a child with autism must do everything correctly to help the child approach normalcy. The child is handicapped in its ability to live and survive. His or her digestive tract and associated organs are so damaged by environmental contaminants that such a child suffers greatly. These problems not only hinder the body from working correctly, but also prevent it from absorbing and processing the nutrients it needs from the foods it consumes.

HEALTH SPEAKS FOR ITSELF

In recent times, a whole new enterprise has arisen that most refer to as "the natural foods and supplement industry". We live in a very market-driven country and, if there is no market for a product, the product does not make it. Well, the fact that the natural foods and supplement industry has mushroomed in the last 50 years or so, and is continuing to grow in an exponential fashion, proves that consuming natural food and supplements help people become healthy and stay healthy. This book provides the evidence of why many of the people in this country have had to shift their focus and pursue becoming healthy eaters and consumers of natural supplements.

PURE FOOD AND SUPPLEMENTS A MUST

The end result of deficient, contaminated soil is that our country's health care costs have skyrocketed while the quality of life has plummeted. (85) For anyone to play blind to these facts is sheer stupidity. The children on whom we have focused this book are the result of this lack of care for our food supply. So they, more than anyone else, need to depend on natural pure food and supplements. An example of the latter are the Ultra-Tested supplements for treating children with autism available from Kirkman Laboratories. (125) Another is Syndion, a multi vitamin, multi mineral, and antioxidant. (126) A third is the omega acids marketed by Nordic Naturals (127) and also by Carlson's. (128) Another supplier I regularly use is Emerson Ecologics (they carry herbs and many quality name brand lines, such as Allergy Research Group, Barlean's, BioRay, BodyBio, Complementary Prescriptions, Designs for Health, Douglas Laboratories, Econugenics, Klaire/Prothera Laboratories who offer prebiotics, probiotics and biofilm products, Metabolic Maintenance, Metagenics, New Chapter/New Mark, Pure Encapsulations. Vital Nutrients, WiseWoman Herbals, and World Nutrition whose enzymes also appear to have anti-biofilm activity). (129) Swanson Vitamins is an option. (130) Thorne Research products are magnesium stearate-free.

AN "A" FOR EFFORT

It is a matter of reality that health care practitioners from psychologists to medical doctors, as well as others who try to help these children all have to focus on what works. They are trying to help these poor children to live semi-normal lives and be able to live at peace with their parents and families.

THE HEALTHIEST, PUREST, FRESHEST FOOD REQUIRED

With this background, I will point out once again that the ideal solution for a family that has a child with autism is to have its own garden and keep its own domestic animals. This will put the family in complete control of the food supply and, as a result, it will be able to produce nutrient-dense and pure food. If this is impossible, for example, for those trapped in cities, the family then has to depend on the best supplements available, as well as on the healthiest, purest, and freshest food it can find. This is the alternative regimen I mentioned above.

BODIES MUST HAVE THE ESSENTIALS

As noted, this means the family should provide the children with autism with the indispensable nutrients which include the essential vitamins, minerals, oils, enzymes, and proteins. All children who suffer from autism and, for that matter, all human beings, must have the essentials or the bodies will "fall apart". And many do these days.

EAT GOOD FOOD, GET RID OF TOXINS

This book is not the place to evaluate all the products available. Suffice it to say each health care practitioner caring for children with autism has his or her favorites. I recommend management include appropriate physical, occupational, and speech therapies. The key point is that all parents must do what they have to do in this regard. They must also have an ongoing detoxification program as discussed in this chapter.

TRACE MINERALS AND SEA PRODUCTS

I will also add, however, that increasing numbers of health care practitioners and parents are not aware of the importance of trace minerals to the body. I strongly recommend that each person who is helping a child with autism in any way read the book by Dr. Brownstein about iodine and its importance in metabolism and detoxification entitled *Iodine-Why you Need It And Why You Can't Live Without It.* (131) They should provide at least a supplement containing products from the sea, such as Super Sea Veg. (132) Readers are urged to visit this web site to learn about the many benefits of sea vegetables. Similar products can also be purchased from Maine Coast Sea Vegetables, preferably one of their formulations containing iodine. (133) Both sources offer small portions of sea vegetables that really are very important foods to add to every person's diet. As stated by Dr. Cabot, sea vegetables not only add many nutrients to the body but also contribute natural substances to help the body rid itself of harmful contaminants. In addition, sea vegetables are pure and free from contamination compared with land-grown crops. Unfortunately, the American public has not been exposed to such foods to the same degree as the people in Japan, Ireland, and other coastal regions. Therefore, everyone should learn about these vital substances by reading one of the many available books about sea vegetables to discover which of these foods need to be introduced into their diet. The many wonderful nutrients available in sea vegetables are presented in Appendix E. This table was used with permission from the book *Sea Vegetable Celebration*.

RESOURCES

The care of a child with autism is far from easy. But, over time with an emphasis on feeding the child "perfect food" and having an ongoing detoxification program, much can be done to help the child. I recommend the detoxification program proposed in the books by Dr. Cabot. I feel it is the best one to help these little canaries to leave their cages and perhaps become normal, productive persons in society.

IT CAN BE DONE

We have the example of this happening in the person of Temple Grandin. I urge all concerned persons to view the film about her and read the books she has written. The parents of children with autism can only do their best. This woman and those who helped her certainly did the best they could and the results were very positive.

Her web site is www.templegrandin.com.

A WHOLE COUNTRY WITHOUT AUTISM

I end this book by returning to those who, for fear of loss of herd immunity and for other reasons, still staunchly advocate a rigorous vaccination schedule. These people should pay special attention to what is occurring in Cuba and the low incidence of autism there. If this data can be validated, the answer may lie in adopting a similar natural soil care program and in restricting the use of acetaminophen-containing medications. Such compounds may be only the tip of the iceberg of medications as potential poisons. A program like those mentioned in this and other books by concerned medical practitioners has the potential to reverse the current autism epidemic. Cuba, a country the size of one of our states, did it --and so can we. All it takes is inspiration, dedication, and determination.

However, to increase the chance for this program to succeed, one thing more is needed:

FOCUS ON LIVER HEALTH

Especially because many children will still develop autism during the transition and implementation period of this endeavor, without delay we must embark on and continue a national program of liver cleansing, support, and protection. Caring for the liver plays a key role in the management and prevention of autism. Nothing can replace this attention.

Nothing less than this will work. Each one of us must accept this truth and change how we think and live. Time is very short now. Our world is becoming more toxic by the second. Not only the lives of children with autism, but *all life* hangs in the balance.

HELP FROM ABOVE

Hopefully, this book has provided some useful information for accomplishing the goals mentioned above. I would also suggest that all turn to prayer and meditation for, with God, *nothing is impossible.* And even if a family has to continue living with a child with severe autism, the family can at least obtain the strength and determination to do as best it can and live a happy, joyful life, a goal which every one of us should strive to achieve.

Epilogue

The Problem Solved

ONLY ONE

Thank you for reading this book. Together we will make a difference. I wanted to do something to stem the scourge of autism. This book is my best shot at it. If one child is saved from autism due to this effort, it will all have been worth it!

WITH LIGHT, DARKNESS DISAPPEARS

Chapter One mentioned a fire truck. This Epilogue returns to the fire truck. When the alarm rings sending fire fighters to a raging blaze, they busy themselves extinguishing it without immediate concern as to how or where the fire began. Autism is an alarming childhood disease that is spreading like a wild fire out of control. Autism is enveloping our world. You and I are the fire fighters. Just as firefighters operate in their domain, our main concern should be to extinguish this fire and hopefully to prevent it from ever developing in the first place. This entails learning how autism originates. The efforts of many have brought to light credible causes and effective management measures. Now they can be appropriately implemented.

WHATEVER HAPPENED TO MY WIFE JILL?

This book began with the story about my wife. Here is some

follow-up information. Since beginning the Liver Cleansing Diet, especially the juicing, Jill has been able to successfully discontinue all her prescription medications within a year. I advise patients not to attempt this without appropriate medical guidance. Her fibromyalgia has improved dramatically. She thinks and remembers more clearly now. Her health is better since we left our home in the suburbs and moved to a small garden farm twelve years ago. Today, Jill is able to work here on Abba's Acres and at times care for all of the animals by herself. She has energy left over for a number of other activities. She has assisted with the editing of this book.

MODEMS AND BIOTOXINS

Although Jill is not 100% better as of this date because she has developed a sensitivity to electromagnetic fields, we know we are going down the right path. We cannot fully explain her general improvement despite this new sensitivity. While acknowledging the great benefit the Liver Cleansing Diet conferred, our current hypothesis is that her negative reaction to electromagnetic fields, particularly those generated by wireless devices as modems and the newer cordless and I-phones, is related to the colonization of biotoxin-producing pathogenic organisms in her intestinal tract following a course of antibiotics. These organisms view strong environmental electrical fields as an attack on their well being and react by escalating the amount and potency of biotoxin they make. We believe it is these biotoxins that are causing her symptoms.

It appears that the antibiotic she took destroyed the oxalate-metabolizing bacterium described in the oxalates section of Chapter Three that normally resides in our G-I tracts and opened the door to colonization with these pathogens. It is known that accumulation of oxalates in the G-I tract make reimplantation with healthy microbiota very difficult. To counteract this, Jill, who has disturbed oxalate metabolism by organic acid testing (see pp 51-53), is on a low oxalate diet and is repleting her intestinal flora with large doses of probiotics that are known to be able to metabolize oxalates. We have addressed the biotoxin toxicity with large, regular doses of broken cell wall chlorella and aged liquid garlic. (134) All wireless devices in our home have been deactivated.

TAKE YOUR SHOES OFF

Earthing or grounding, such as walking barefoot (especially in the water along a beach) or even lying on the ground outside provide some temporary, symptomatic relief. (135)

FERMENTATION TO THE RESCUE

We found that her unusually high magnesium requirement responded to eating fermented foods, such as sauerkraut and fermented beans and rice. Preparing food in this fashion is known to remove many anti-nutrients that prevent our body from properly using minerals and other essentials in our food. (136) It also responded, we believe, to the elimination of magnesium stearate that was present in the magnesium supplement (see Chapter Three).

We appreciate the great good Drs. Dietrich Klinghardt and Joseph Mercola have brought about by making information which contributed to our hypothesis accessible on Dr. Mercola's website.

ADDITIONAL HELP

If you are suffering with problems similar to Jill's, especially fibromyalgia and environmental sensitivity, I suggest you also read Dr. Cabot's books, review the chlorella information on the website noted above, and obtain two very helpful papers by Dr. Stephen Genuis. (137,138)

Jill still has her ups and downs, but she certainly has made progress by following a lifestyle of less environmental contamination, and by living on a small family garden farm and keeping animals. Without question, following the Liver Cleansing Diet and juicing have been key to her improvement.

EXCELLENT RESOURCES

Will my recommendations presented in this book be effective in combating the autism epidemic? I believe they will, based on a lifestyle noted above and described throughout this book, following an individualized immunization program, waging a winning battle against the Enemy Within and the Enemy Without, and implementing the Liver Cleansing Diet.

WE HAVE PURPOSE AND GOALS TO PURSUE

Will these changes be easy for you to make for yourself and your child? Probably not. Will they work for your child? Although there are few certainties in life, I feel there is much hope for success by putting the concepts presented in these pages into practice. Which tests will be needed to assess the liver function of newborns is a matter for experts to determine. This matter needs to be settled post haste.

IN CLOSING

In the meantime, let us move forward with the knowledge we already possess. We have been marking time for too long. We must change for the better. Hopefully, you will agree with the pathway proposed in these pages, and, as a consequence, soon begin all these measures for the sake of your child's well-being as well as for your own.

May God bless your efforts and reward your child and you with the health you so earnestly seek and, for all your hard work, greatly deserve!

References

1. Bouquot JE, McMahon RE. Ischemic osteonecrosis in facial pain syndromes; a review of NICO (neuralgia-inducing cavitational osteonecrosis) based on experience with more than 2,000 patients. *TM Diary* 1996;8:32-39.

2. Liska D. Development of the knowledge base in biochemical individuality. In: Jones DS, Quinn S, eds. *Textbook of Functional Medicine.* Gig Harbor, WA: Institute for Functional Medicine;2005:63-75.

3. Liska D, Lyon M, Jones DS. Detoxification and Biotransformational Imbalances. In reference (2):277.

4. Cabot S. *The Healthy Liver and Bowel Book*. 4th ed. Glendale, AZ: SCB International Inc; 1999:15-16.

5. McGinnis WR. Oxidative stress in autism. In reference (2):512-516

6. Hyman M. The matrix: dietary influences on oxidative stress, mitochondrial function, and energy metabolism. In reference (2):362-363.

7. Reference (4):15-16.

8. Pangborn J. Overview of the Defeat Autism Now biomedical approach. Presented at: Autism Research Institute DAN! Defeat Autism Now Meeting; ober 23-26, 2008; San Diego, CA.

9. Null, G. Vaccine Nation. [DVD]. New York, NY; Gary Null & Associates, Inc; 2008. http://vaccinenation.net. Accessed June 25, 2012.

10. Manookian L, Nelson K, Pilaro C *The Greater Good.* A documentary film. Hailey ID: BNP Pictures, LLC; 2011.[DVD]. http://www.greater good movie.org/home. Accessed June 25, 2012.

11. Williams R. *Biochemical Individuality*. New York, NY: John Wiley and Sons; 1956.

12. Recommended immunization schedules for persons aged 0 through 18 years—United States, 2011. MMWR. 2011;60:1-4. In *JAMA*. May 25, 2011; 305(20):2062-2065.

13. *Physicians Desk Reference* 66th ed. 2012. Montvale, NJ:1901 Used with permission of the PDR Network, LLC. Publisher of *Physicians' Desk Reference*. PDR Network, LLC.209, p36. All Rights Reserved.

14. Landis J. Drugs and theelderly. http://www.tje hospitalist.org/details/article/234051/Drugs_and_the_Elderly.html. Accessed June 25, 2012.

15. Cave S, Mitchell D. *What Your Doctor May Not Tell You About Childhood Vaccinations*. revised ed. New York: Wellness Central; 2010. Also available in E-form.

16. Sears RW. *The Vaccine Book.* New York, NY: Little Brown and Company; 2007.

17. Cave S. Vaccine update for parents and professionals. Presented at: Autism Research Institute DAN! Defeat Autism Now Conference; April 19-23; 2007; Alexandria, VA.

18. Olmsted D, Blaxill M. *The Age of Autism.* New York, NY: St. Marten's Press; 2010:241,282-283.

19. http://www.NVIC.org. Accessed June 25, 2012.

20. Reference (18):252-254.

21. Buie T, Campbell DB, Fuchs GJ 3rd, et al. Evaluation, diagnosis, and treatment of gastrointestinal disorders in individuals with ASDs: a consensus report. *Pediatrics.* Jan 2010;125(suppl1):S1-18.

22. Buie T, Fuchs GJ 3rd, Furuta G, et al. Recommendations for evaluation and treatment of common gastrointestinal problems in children with ASDs. *Pediatrics*. Jan 2010;125(suppl1):S19-29.

23. Olmstead S, Snodgrass R, Meiss D, Ralston J. Micrometabolic imprinting in infancy: miroflora, probiotics, and chronic disease. Klaire Labs Technical Summary. 2007. PDF Access article using first author and title. Accessed June 25 2012.

24. Olszak T, An D, Zeissig S, et al. Microbial exposure during early life has persistent effects on natural killer T cell function. *Science* 27 April 2012;336(6080):489-493. In *JAMA.* May 2, 2012;307(17):1790.

25. Should auld acquaintance be forgot... - NCBI - NIH. Accessed June 25, 2012.

26. Hanaway P. Balance of flora, GALT, and mucosal integrity. In reference (2): 444-453.

27. Olmstead S, Meiss D, Ralston J. Life on the edge: the clinical implications of gastrointestinal biofilm. Klaire Labs Technical Summary. 2009. http://www.medspane.com/files/43870640.pdf Accessed 25 June, 2012.

28. Sult T. Organisms of the gut. In reference (2):332-333.

29. Gottschall E. *Breaking The Vicious Cycle: Intestinal Health Through Diet.* Baltimore, Ontario, Canada: Kirkton Press; 2004:8, 45-49

30. Krigsman A, Boris M, Goldblatt A, Stott C. Clinical presentation and histologic findings at ileocolonoscopy in children with autistic spectrum disorder and chronic gastrointestinal symptoms. (epub prior to print publicat). In *Autism Research Review Inernational.* 2010;24(1):1.

31. Sult T. Clinical approaches to Gastrointestinal Imbalance:Heavy Metals. In reference (2):440.

32. Cave S. Detoxification & autism spectrum disorders. Presented at: GI Detoxification: Probiotics, Enzymes, and Complementary Agents Meeting; November 13-14, 2009; Salt Lake City, UT.

33. Lin HC. Small intestinal bacterial overgrowth, a framework for understanding irritable bowel syndrome. *JAMA.* Aug 18, 2004; 292:852-858.

34. Cabot S, Jasinska M. *The Ultimate Detox.* Camden, NSW, AU. WHAS; 2005: 52-53,74-77.

35. Fasano A. Surprises from celiac disease. *Scientific American.* Aug 2009:54-61.

36. Delzenne N, Cani P. Probiotics and Prebiotics. Presented in: *Functional Medicine Update.* August 2009. Puyallup WA. *Synthesis* by Jeffey Bland PhD.

Brncik C. Jun 19, 2011. http://www.livestrong.com/article/47442-can-

37. http://www.food-allergies cause-swelling-in...Accessed June 25, 2012.

38. Coca A. *The Pulse Test.* In: Hygiene Library Catalog. http://www. soiland health.org. Accessed June 25, 2012.

39. Konstantynowicz J, Porowski T, Zoch-Zwierz W, et al. A potential pathogenic role of oxalates in autism. European Journal of Paediatric Neurology (2011),doi:10.1016/j.ejpn.2011.08.004 Accessed June 25, 2012.

40. http://lowoxalate.info/papers/mechanisms.html. Accessed June 25, 2012.

41. http: www.lowoxalate.info/. Accessed June 25, 2012.

42. Baker SM. Gluten-and Casein-Free Diets. In: Pangborn J, Baker SM. *Autism: Effective Biomedical Treatments.* San Diego, CA: Autism Research Institute:2005:104-108, 110-111.

43. Gershon MD. *The Second Brain.* New York, NY: Harper Collins Publishers: 1998.

44. O'Bryan T. *Unlocking the Mystery of Wheat & Gluten Sensitivity.* 2006 [DVD]. Also: *Identifying and Conquering Gluten Sensitivity – Inside and outside the gut.* [DVD]. http://www.theDr.com (products). Accessed June 25, 2012.

45. Barcia G, Posar A, Santucci M, et al. Autism and celiac disease. *J Autism Dev Disord:* 38:407-408.

46. Di Sabatino A, Corazza GR. Nonceliac gluten sensitivity: sense or sensibility? Ann Int Med:Feb 21, 2012;156(4):309-311.

47. Pangborn J. Methionine Metabolism. In reference (42):162.

48. Rossignol DA. Novel and emerging treatments for autism spectrum disorders: a systematic review. *Ann Clin Psychiatry.* November, 2009; 21(4):220-221.

49. Lukaczer D. The "4-R" Program. In reference (2):462-468.

50. Welch MG, Anwar M, Chang CY, et al. Combined administration of secretin and oxytocin inhibits chronic colitis and associated activation of forebrain neurons. *Neurogastroenterol Motil.* June 2010;22(6):654-e202*

51. Olmert MD. *Made For Each Other. The biology of the human-animal bond.* Philadelphia, PA: Da Capo Press; 2009.

52. Herbert MR. Autism, biology, and the environment. Autism is treatable: scientific plausibility. Presented at: Autism Research Institute DAN! Defeat Autism Now Meeting. Apr 7-10, 2006; Washington, DC.

53. Environmental Working Group. The Body Burden: the pollution in newborns, a benchmark investigation of industrial chemicals, pollutants, and pesticides in human umbilical cord blood. Jul 21, 2005. www.ewg.org/reports/body burden2Accessed June 25, 2012.

54. Herbert MR. How the environment interfaces with the whole body; chronic, and treatable features of neurodevelopmental disorders: the case of autism . Presented at: 2011 Conference on Environmental Toxicity and Neurodevelopmental Disorders. June 24, 2011. Duquense Univeristy. Pittsburgh PA.

55. Mesnage R, Clair E, Gress S, et al. Cytotoxicity on human cells of CRY1Ab and CRY1Ac Bt insecticidal toxins alone or with a glyphosate-based herbicide. *J Appl Toxicol.* First published on line February 15,2012. DOI: 10.1002/jat2712. Accessed June 25, 2012.56

56. Koller VJ, Furhacker M, Nersesyan A, et al. Cytotoxic and DNA-damaging properties of glyphosate and Roundup® in human-derived buccal epithelial cells. Arch Toxicol. Feb 14, 2012. http://www.ncbi.nlm.nih.gov/Pubmed/22331240. Accessed Jun 25, 2012.

57. Benachour N, Seralini DE. Glyphosate formulations induce apoptosis and necrosis in human umbilical, embryonic, and placental cells. Chem Res Toxicol. 2009; 22(1):97-105.

58. Huber, D. Side Effects of Glyphosate on Soil and Nutrients. Presented at: BioAg Seminar Jan 19, 2011. BioAg Consultants and Distributors, Inc. 1400 Greenwood Hill Rd. Wellesley, ON. NOB 250 Canada. (800)363-5278. Http://www.bio-ag.com. Accessed June 25, 2012.

59. Wallace H. Foreward. *Soils and Men.Yearbook of Agriculture 1938.* Washington, DC. USDA. United States Government Printing Office. 1938:v.

60. Landrigan P. The exquisite vulnerability of the developing human brain to toxic chemicals in the environment. Presented at: 2011

Conference on Environmental Toxicity and Neurodevelopmental Disorders. Jun 24, 2011 Duquense University. Pittsburgh, PA.

61. Carson, R. *Silent Spring*. Boston, MA. Houghton Mifflin; 1962.

62. http://www.epa.gov/tri/triprogram/whatis.htm. Accessed 25 June, 2012

63. CDC. Prevalence of Autism Spectrum Disorders – Autism and Developmental Disabilities Monitoring Network, 14 States, United States, 2008. MMWR 2012:61(No. SS-3):1-19.

64. Kaplan S. Reform of Toxic Chemicals Law Collapses as Industry Flexes Its Muscles. www.politicsdaily.com/.../risky-business-epa-builds- list-of-potentially-dangerous-chemicals.12/21/10. Accessed June 25, 2012.

65. The UN Millenium Ecosystem Assessment. http://www.publications.parlament.uk/pa/cm200607/cmselect/.../77.pdf. Accessed June 25, 2012.

66. Dindyal S. 2004. http://www.ispub.com/journal/.../internet-journal-of-urology/.../the-sperm-c... Accessed 25 June, 2012.

67. http://en.wikipedia.org/wiki/Total-fertility-rate. Accessed June 25, 2012.

68. Cho SC, Bhang SY, Hong Y C, et al. Relationship between environmental phthalate exposure and the intelligence of school-aged children. *Environ Health Perspectives.* Jul 2010; 118(7):1027-32.

69. Wallis C. Study in Korea puts autism's prevalence at 2.6%, surprising experts. *New York Times*. May 9, 2011.

70. Mutler A, Jahn G. A-P October 11, 2010. Communism left Toxic Legacy in Eastern Europe. Http://www.boston.com/.../Europe/2010/communism-left-toxic-legac. Accessed June 25, 2012.

71. Welch MG, Klein BY. Possible mechanism involving intestinal oxytocin, oxidative stress, and signaling pathways in a subset of autism with gut symptoms. In: *Autism, Oxidative Stress, Inflammation, and Immune Abnormalities*. New York, NY: Taylor & Francis. CRC Press; 2010:299-314.

72. Rutter DO. A growing concern: hazardous waste in fertilizer. www.newfarm.rodaleinstitute.org/depts/gleanings/0803/rutter.shtml

Accessed June 25, 2012.

73. International Ag Labs. A biological approach to agriculture . 800 Lake Avenue. Fairmont, MN 56031. Ph. 507 235 6909. http://www.aglabs.com and http://highbrixgardens.com. Accessed June 25, 2012.

74. Sorensen E. EPA to hold hearings on waste in fertilizer. Seattle Times. November 28, 2001.

75. Rosenkranz HS, Anderson MD. Identification and action of environmental carcinogens. *HAMA'ABADA* (*J of the Israel Biochem and Microbiol Assoc*) January, 1973;(1):70-84.

76. *Captan Health and safety Guide.* No. 50. Geneva SW. Pub. 390. WHO.1990; Item 2.3.

77. Haley B. Thimerosal, mercury, and neurological impairment at the molecular level. Presented at: Autism Research Institute DAN! Defeat Autism Now Meeting. October 1-3, 2004. Los Angeles, CA.

78. Pusztai, A. The Dangers of GMO's. Presented at: BioAg Seminar. January 19, 2011. See ref. (58).

79. Aris A, Leblanc S. Maternal and fetal exposure to pesticides are associated to genetically modified foods in Eastern townships of Quebec, Canada. *Reprod Toxicol.* May 31, 2011;(4):528-533.

80. Peavy W, Peary W. *Super Nutrition Gardening. How to grow your own supercharged food.* Garden City Park, NY: Avery Publishing Co;1993:3

81. Luebke S, Luebke U. *Pioneers of Microbial Composting.* Peuerbach , Austria. http://www.ibiblio.org/steved/Luebke/Luebke-compost2.html. Accessed June 25, 2012.

82. Musilova J, Bystricka J, Vollmannova A, Melichacova S, et al Contamination of potato tubers by heavy metals and their influence in the formation of phenol substances. *J of Central Eur Agriculture.* 2011;12(3):433-444.

83. Angelova V, Ivanova R, Pevicharova G Ivanov K. Effect of organic amendments of heavy metal uptake by potato plants. Presented at:

World Congress of Soil Science; soil solutions for a changing world. Aug 1-6, 2010; Brisbane, Australia.

84. Werner M. Cuba's Composting! Http://www.fadr.msu.ru/rodale/agsieve/txt/vol7/art1.html. Accessed June 25, 2012.

85. Howard A. *An Agricultural Testament.* London, UK: Humphrey Milford; and New York, NY: Oxford University Press. 1940. Republished by Oxford City Press in 2010: 5-25, 184-193.

86. Shaw, W. Unraveling the Cause of the Autism Epidemic. Online webinar. Jan 11, 2012. Great Plains Laboratory. Lanexa KA. http://www.greatplains laboratory.com. Publication pending. See: http;//wwwimmunizationprofile/cuba/who , http://www.immunizationprofile/unitedstatesofamerica/who, and Tocco M. Side Effects of Acetaminophen. Jan 11, 2012. http://www. childhood shots.com/Adverse-Side-Effects-of-Acetaminophen-s/196.htm. All sites accessed June 25, 2012.

87. Gempler's. P.O. Box 44993. Madison, WI. 53744-4993. 800-382-8473. In: product support at: http://www.gemplers.com. Accessed June 25, 2012.

88. Muhammad A. Cuba, the Compost King. http://lifeabundantly-alim.blogspot.com/2010/05/cuba-compost-king-.html. Accessed June 25,2012.

89. Reference (61):22, 18-80

90. Schlosser, E. *Fast Food Nation: The dark side of the American meal.* Boston-New York:Mariner Books Houghton Miflfin:2012:45. Quoted from: Acuff DS. *What Kids Eat and Why.* New York:Simon &Schuster:1997.

91. Animal Assisted Therapy Day Jun 11, 2011. Held at: PEACE Ranch. Professional Equine Assisted Counseling & Education. Kaschel, J. executive director. 2566 Hoosier Valley Rd. Traverse City, MI 49684. http:wwwpeaceranchtc.com. E-mail: peaceranchtc @gmail.com. Website and E-mail accessed June 25, 2012.

92. Psalm 13:2 (Ps.130 in some versions).

93. Popper DE, Popper FJ. An America without Farmers? Apr 8, 2004. In: publications; prairie writers circle at http://www.landinstitute.org/ Accessed June 25, 2012.

94. Reference (35): 32.

95.Cabot S. *The Liver Cleansing Diet.* Glendale, AZ: SCB International; 1997:34,50-52.

96. Reference (34):17-25.

97. Reference (95):7-11, 25-37.

98. Reference (4):7-10, 63.

99. Reference (95):81-83.

100. Reference (95):50.

101. Reference (34):30-31.

102. Reference (4):7, 12-16.

103.Reference (95):45-46.

104. Reference (95):28,29

105. Reference (4):36-38.

106. Reference (95):92-93.

107. Cabot S. *Fatty Liver You Can Reverse It.* Glendale AZ; SCB Inc. International; 2010:15-22.

108. Rice, C. Summary of Workshop on Evaluating Change in ASD Prevalence. February, 2011.http://www.iacc.hhs.gov/events/slides -cathy-rice-041111.pdf. Accessed June 25, 2012.

109. Hallmayer, J, Cleveland S, Torres, A, et al. Genetic heritability and shared environmental factors among twin pairs with autism. *Arch Gen Psychiatry.* 2011;68(1):1095-1102. See also: Digitale E. Non-genetic factors play surprisingly large role in determining autism, says study by group. http://www.med. stanford.edu/ism/2011/july/autism.html. Accessed June 25, 2012.

110. Poultry drug sales suspended. *JAMA,* July 13, 2011;306(2):143. tinyurl.com/3dcj5y9. Accessed June 25, 2012.

111. Dioxin Advisory Information. In: http://www.michigan.gov/hunting/ antlerless deer hunting digest. Accessed June 25, 2012.

112. Steinman D. *Diet For a Poisoned Planet,* New York, NY:Harmony Books, 1990:89-93

113. Reference (61):15.

114. Reference (34):12.

115. Shanahan C, Shanahan L. *Deep Nutrition Why your genes need traditional food.* Lawai, HI: Big Box Books; 2009:3-5

116. Reference (2):73.

117. Reference (4):17-19.

118. Vaccination of Persons with Primary and Secondary Immune Deficiencies. http://www.cdc.gov/vaccines/pubs/ pinkbook/ downloads/appendices/A/immuno-table.pdf. Accessed June 25, 2012.

119. Campbell McBride N. *Gut and Psychology Syndrome. Cambridge,* UK:Medinform Publishing; 2004:61

120. Gellen BG, Mailbach EK, Marcuse EK Do parents understand immunizations? A national telephone survey *Pediatrics.* November 1, 2000;106(5);1097-1102.

121. Immunization Safety Review: Multiple Immunizations and Immune Dysfunction. McCormick M. chair. Institute of Medicine. February 20, 2002:4,17. http://www.lom.edu/Reports/2002/ Immunization-Safety-Review-Multiple-Immunizations. Accessed June 25, 2012.

122. Kuehn B. IOM Review Finds Vaccine Adverse Events Are Rare and Usually Reversible. *JAMA* 2011; 306(13);1427-1428. doi:10.1001/jama.2011.1386. Accessed June 25, 2012.

123. Reference (95):12-14

124. Price-Pottinger Nutrition Foundation, Inc. 7890 Broadway Lemon Grove, CA,91945 http://www.ppnf.org. E-mail: info@ppnf.org. Also: Price- Pottinger Journal of Health and Healing. Accessed June 25, 2012.

125. Kirkman. 6400 S.W. Rosewood St. Lake Oswego, OR 97035. (800) 245- 8282. www.kirkmanlabs.com. Accessed June25, 2012.

126. Yasoo Health Products. 2109 W. Market Street, Suite 154 Johnson City, TN 37604-0024 (888)469-2766. http://www.yasooproducts.com/syndion/supplement.html. Accessed June 25, 2012

127. Nordic Naturals, Inc. Watsonville, CA 95076. (800)662-2544 http://www.nordicnaturals.com/ Accessed June 25, 2012.

128. Carlson Nutritional Supplements. http://www.carlsonlabs.com/ (888)234 5656. Accessed June 25, 2012.

129. Emerson Ecologics. 7 Commerce Drive. Bedford, NH 03110. (800) 654 432. www.emersonecologics.com/Accessed. June 25, 2012.

130. Swanson Health Products. Box 2803, Fargo, ND 58108-2803. (800) 437 4148. www.swansonvitamins.com Accessed June 25, 2012.

131. Brownstein D. *Iodine Why You Need It. Why you can't live without it.* 4th ed. West Bloomfield, MI. Medical Alternative Press 2009. http://www.drbrownstein.com/ Accessed June 25, 2012.

132. Farma Sea ® Health, LLC. (800) 893-8344. http://www.farmasea. Com Accessed June 25, 2012.

133. Maine Coast Sea Vegetables 3 Georges Pond Rd., Franklin, ME 04634. (207)565 2907. wwww.seaveg.com. Accessed June 25, 2012.

134. The Klinghardt Neurotoxin Elimination protocol. Http://www.hbci.com/~wenonah/new/9steps.htm. Accessed June 25, 2012.

135. Earthing. http://www.earthing.com/ Accessed June 25, 2012.

136. Hunter BT. *Probiotic Foods for Good Health. Yogurt,sauerkraut, and other beneficial fermented foods.* 2008.Laguna Beach, CA. Basic Health Publishers, Inc:143.

137. Genuis SJ. Sensitivity-related illness: The escalating pandemic of allergy, food intolerance, and chemical sensitivity. Http://www.aipro.info/drive/File/Sensitivity- Accessed June 25, 2012.

138. Genuis SJ. Fielding a current idea: exploring the public health impact of electromagnetic radiation. *Public Health* (2007).: DOI: 10.1016/j.puhe.2007.04 008. Accessed June 25, 2012.

Resource Laboratories Referred to in This Book

Applied Isotope Technologies, Inc. 2403 Sidney St. Suite 280 Pittsburgh, PA 15203. (412) 223-2096. http://sidms.com

Doctor's Data, Inc. 3755 Illinois Ave. St. Charles, IL 60174-2420. (800) 323-2784 www.Doctorsdata.com

Genova Diagnostics. 63 Zilicoa Street. Ashville, NC 28801. 800-522-2762. www.gdx.net

Great Plains Laboratory. 11813 W. 77th St. Lenexa, KS 66214. 913-341-8949. www.greatplainslaboratory.com

Metametrix Clinical Lab, 3425 Corporate Way, Duluth, GA 30096 (800) 221-4640

Appendix A

Pediatric Exposure to Several Medications Raises Safety Concerns

News Author: Kate Johnson

01/05/2012 Reprinted from Medscape education Clinical Briefs. (used with permission)

Clinical Context

Iatrogenic complications can be more serious among children vs adults, and the inpatient setting presents an especially high risk for drug errors, adverse effects, and interactions among children. A previous review of a large database of pediatric inpatients by Lasky and colleagues, which was published in the January 2011 issue of *Pharmacoepidemiology and Drug Safety,* found that acetaminophen was the most commonly prescribed medication during hospitalization, followed by lidocaine, ampicillin, gentamicin, and fentanyl.

The current study by Feudtner and colleagues further examines the use of medications among hospitalized children, particularly regarding trends in polypharmacy in comparing different hospital settings, patient ages, and conditions.

Study Synopsis and Perspective

A large proportion of hospitalized children are exposed to numerous medications on a daily basis in both children's and general hospitals throughout the United States, according to a new study by Chris Feudtner, MD, PhD, from the University of Pennsylvania School of Medicine, Philadelphia, and colleagues.

In addition, children with rare conditions are more likely to be exposed to more substantial polypharmacy, the authors report in an article published in the January issue of the *Archives of Pediatric and Adolescent Medicine*.

The findings raise patient safety concerns, "given the relationship between polypharmacy and adverse drug events that has been documented for adults in both hospital and nursing home settings," the authors write, and warrants further investigation into drug–drug interactions.

The study used 2006 data from 2 sources: the Pediatric Health Information System, which comprises administrative discharge data from children's hospitals for most US major metropolitan areas, and the Perspective Data Warehouse, which comprises data from academic medical centers, community-based hospitals, and large hospital systems in both rural and urban settings.

In total, the data included 491,451 pediatric hospitalizations in 52 children's hospitals and 260,740 pediatric hospitalizations in 411 general hospitals, representing nearly one fifth of all pediatric hospitalizations across the country for 2006.

"The total number of drug and therapeutic agent exposures over the course of the entire hospitalization equaled a dozen drugs and therapeutic agents for the typical patient admitted to a children's hospital (with a median LOS [length of stay] of 5 days)," they report, "but was only 2 drugs and therapeutic agents for the typical patient admitted to a general hospital (with a median LOS of 2 days)."

This represents exposure of children in children's hospitals to 1.34 times more drugs and therapeutic agents than children admitted to general hospitals, but after adjustment for patient age, sex, LOS, whether surgery was performed, and rarity of medical condition (All Patient Refined Diagnostic Related Groups), the exposure difference between types of hospital is nullified, the authors note.

The study found that for infant patients (younger than 12 months), the typical (median) exposure on the first day of hospitalization in a children's hospital was 4 distinct generic drugs and therapeutic agents; for infants in the 90th percentile of exposure, it was 11.

For children aged 12 months or older, the median and 90th percentile exposures on the first day of hospitalization were 5 and 13 exposures, respectively.

For patients whose LOS reached 30 days, typical and 90th percentile exposures for infants reached 4 and 13, respectively, by 30 days, whereas patients 1 year or older had 9 and 20 exposures, respectively.

The cumulative number of distinct generic drug and therapeutic agent exposures for each successive day of hospitalization was 25 (median) and 51 (90th percentile) for infants, and 42 (median) and 66 (90th percentile) for older children in children's hospitals.

The highest level of cumulative exposure was for patients with less common conditions. Exposure varied considerably between hospitals among patients with the most common conditions of asthma, appendectomy, and seizure, the authors report.

Although the data displayed initial differences between children's hospitals and general hospitals, adjustment for patient case mix showed that this difference was largely explained by differences in patient populations.

"[W]e found that the most common generic drugs and therapeutic agents to which children were exposed included intravenous fluids; analgesics such as the narcotics fentanyl and morphine or the antipyretics/analgesics acetaminophen and ibuprofen; anti-infective agents such as ampicillin, gentamicin, and cephalosporins; anesthetic agents such as lidocaine and propofol; gastrointestinal drugs such as ranitidine, ondansetron, and metoclopramide; and a bundle of drugs often provided to newborns as part of routine care, including vitamin K, erythromycin eye drops, immunization drugs, and application of triple dye anti-infective agents to the umbilicus," the authors write.

“Exposure to certain classes of drugs such as antineoplastic and cardiovascular agents were much more likely to occur in children's hospitals,” they add.

In an editorial accompanying the article, Nancy Morden, MD, and David Goodman, MD, from the Dartmouth Medical School in Lebanon, New Hampshire, write: "We share the authors' unease with the level of polypharmacy in pediatric inpatient settings, but our biggest concern is the lack of information that would tell us if these prescribing patterns are problematic for patients."

Although evidence suggests that complex medication combinations increase the risk for adverse drug events, there is a need to balance this risk with the benefits of symptom relief or disease modification, the editorialists note. "[T]he tragic undertreatment of pain in children has been extensively documented. In addition, the use of anesthetics and sedatives may not be optional when surgery, procedures, or advanced imaging are required.”

An important next step is to measure outcomes associated with exposure patterns, they add.

Finally, although pediatric polypharmacy is likely most common in the hospitalized patient, "outpatient polypharmacy is increasingly prevalent in children and also deserves attention."

"Therapy with medications started in childhood for management of chronic conditions often continues for decades — well beyond the duration of any drug approval trials and thus well outside our understanding of potential drug effects," the editorialists conclude.

The study was supported by a Center for Education and Research on Therapeutics grant from the Agency for Healthcare Research and Quality. The study authors and Dr. Morden have disclosed no relevant financial relationships. Dr. Goodman currently receives research funding through grants and contracts from the Robert Wood Johnson Foundation; Health Resources and Services Administration; Department of

Health and Human Services, Office of the Assistant Secretary of Planning and Evaluation; National Institute on Aging; National Cancer Institute; and Wellpoint Foundation, and during the last 3 years he has accepted speaker and consulting fees for a number of companies, hospitals, and agencies, a full list of which is available in the article.

Arch Pediatr Adolesc Med. 2012;166:9-16.

Study Highlights

- Researchers used 2 data systems to obtain their study information, and they focused on pediatric admissions among individuals younger than 18 years during 2006. The Pediatric Health Information System provided data from children's hospitals, and the Perspective Data Warehouse includes information from multiple types of hospitals across the United States.
- The study focused on the cumulative use of medications by pediatric inpatients as well as the use of specific medications. Researchers compared medication use according to the type of hospital (children's vs general hospitals), patient age, and diagnosis.
- 365,868 pediatric patients with a total of 491,451 hospitalizations were monitored from children's hospitals, along with 221,559 patients with 260,740 hospitalizations in general hospitals.
- Most children were younger than 4 years, and slightly less than half were white. The average length of hospitalization was 2 to 3 days.
- In children's hospitals, the most common prescription among children younger than 1 year was heparin, and acetaminophen was the most common medication used among children from ages 1 to 9 years. Ondansetron was the common prescription among children and adolescents between the ages of 10 and 17 years.

- In general hospitals, the most commonly used prescriptions (in order) were ampicillin, vitamin K, erythromycin, gentamicin, and acetaminophen.
- Infants and patients 1 year or older were exposed to an average of 3 and 5 drugs on day 1 of hospitalization in general hospitals. The respective values in children's hospitals were 4 and 5 medications.
- On examination of children at the 90th percentile of medication exposure in children's hospitals, infants received an average of 11 drugs on hospital day 1, and older children received an average of 13 drugs. The respective values among children in general hospitals were 8 and 12 medications.
- By day 7, the cumulative average drug exposure was between 22 and 35 medications, depending on patient age and hospital setting.
- Children with less common diagnoses had higher rates of cumulative drug exposure.
- There was substantial heterogeneity in the mean cumulative exposure to medications based on patients' diagnoses, with no trend dependent on the number of pediatric patients treated with that particular diagnosis.
- After adjustment for all patient factors, including diagnosis and length of hospitalization, there was no significant difference in comparing the average number of medications prescribed in children's and general hospitals.

Clinical Implications

- A previous study by Lasky and colleagues of pediatric inpatients found that acetaminophen was the most commonly prescribed medication.
- The current study by Feudtner and colleagues suggests that polypharmacy in hospitalized children is common in both children's and general hospitals. Although children with rare conditions received higher numbers of medications, the number of children treated in the hospital did not affect rates of polypharmacy.

Appendix B

Why Does New Jersey Have the Nation's Second Highest Rate of Autism? A Hypothesis.

In 2006, the New Jersey General Assembly created a legislative package in prompt response to a sobering report released a month prior by the federal Centers for Disease Control and Prevention (CDC). The CDC study found New Jersey to have the nation's highest reported rate of autism –1 out of every 94 children. The national rate at that time was 1 out of 110 children. In 2002, the national rate was 1 out of 150 children. Since autism is a predominately male disease, the 2006 data indicated one in every 58 boys in NJ would be diagnosed with autism, for unclear reasons. (1)

A more recent report shows a worsening picture. Autism rates continue to soar nationwide and New Jersey remains near the top of the list. According to our government's Centers for Disease Control and Prevention (CDC) data released in March, 2012, roughly two percent of children in NJ –or about 1 in 50—will be diagnosed with autism. This study was in 2008. One in 88 children nationwide is believed to have autism or a related disorder. In New Jersey, the rate was 1 in 49, second highest in the nation behind Utah where the rate was 1 in 47.(2)

What has happened to the autism rate since 2008? Recall that the national rate in 2002 was 1 out of 150. In 2006 it was one 1 of 110. In 2008 it jumped to one in 88. But in New Jersey in

2008 it was one in 49 in boys and girls combined. What might it be in 2012, given that this rate of increase shows no signs of leveling off ? And, since autism is fivefold more common in boys, what would be the chances of autism developing in a little boy living in New Jersey today?

NJ cities are not ranked among the nation's ten dirtiest. (3) Yet, a strong link appears to exist between the rate of autism and environmental contamination and autism and the environment. (4) Therefore, a unique environmental etiologic agent may be operative in NJ and awaiting identification and correction. The following hypothesis addresses that puzzle.

For most of the last century, northeastern New Jersey was a center for chromate and bichromate chemical manufacturing. Chromite ore was shipped to two Jersey City facilities and to another nearby facility from around the world. The chromate production process produced about 1.5 lbs of a mud-like residue for every pound of chromium product resulting in an estimated accumulation of between 2 and 3 million tons of processing residue from 1905 to 1976. In 1991 Thomas Burke of the Johns Hopkins School of Hygiene and Public Health was the principal author of a report describing extensive environmental contamination of Hudson County, NJ with this processing residue. Chromium, a known lung cancer causing agent, was present in about 5% of the residue distributed over 130 chromium-contaminated sites, predominately in Jersey City. This residue was sold or given away for use of fill material (including wetlands) and was widely used in construction at residential, commercial, and industrial sites throughout the county. (5)

The New Jersey Department of Health evaluated children and adults with possible exposure to chromium from contaminated fill dirt used in residential areas. School age-children living closest to known chromium-containing sites were more likely to have urine chromium levels above the selected detection limit than children living in zones more distant from known contamination. Boys were more likely to have detectable urine chromium levels. An outdoor exposure to chromium through ingestion or inhalation was postulated. (5)

In Bergen County in December, 1983 approximately 3,640 gallons of chromium plating solution containing 5,441 lbs of chromium were discharged from a partially below ground storage tank. Monitoring wells indicated the presence of ground water contamination with chromium and hexavalent chromium, or chromium (VI), in amounts 15,000 times higher than allowable in federal drinking water standards. A report describing this event by the New Jersey Department of Health and Senior Services states this runoff material likely seeped into moraine deposits and bedrock aquifers from the electroplating site where the discharge occurred. (6)

The crux of the problem is the amount of hexavalent chromium, i.e. chromium (VI), present in situations of environmental contaminations, such as the above two citations. Chromium (VI) is water-soluble, corrosive, causes allergies, genetic mutations, and cancer. It is by far the most toxic and reactive form of chromium. (5)

Conventional analytic methods are reported to underestimate the amount of chromium (VI) in soil residues by about 40% because they are unable to correct for conversion of chromium (VI) to another form, trivalent chromium, or chromium (III), which occurs during analytic procedures currently being used in commercial laboratories, as well as in soil in the natural environment. (7) Sites in NJ containing residue from processed chromite ore contain very high levels of chromium III that is generally regarded to have low toxicity and even occurs naturally. Cleanup action level in NJ is largely directed by the demonstrated presence of chromium (III). However, remediation needs to be based on the finding of biologically damaging chromium (VI) in all that yellow powder that reports show covering the ground at former chemical manufacturing sites. (7) Finding even a 40% increase in chromium (VI) in a site may be sufficient to direct remedial attention to it.

A new, more accurate analytic method, known as United States Environmental Protection Agency Method (USEPA) 6800A is available, which uses speciated isotope dilution mass spectrometry (SIDMS). It is an expensive assay, but with increasing use costs should moderate. This method accurately takes into account, controls for, and corrects interspecies conversion between the chromiums (VI) and (III) occurring during measurement. Experimental studies performed in a number of laboratories comparing the USEPA 6800A method with detection methods currently being used in commercial laboratories corroborate and consistently demonstrate that method 6800A yields levels of chromium (VI) which are approximately 40% higher than commercial methods report and on which current remediation strategies are largely based. (7) However, powerful business and political interests always work vigorously to oppose any measure that would increase responsibility for damage to both man and environment, necessitate further remediation (even re-remediation) and interfere with economic development of their region. (8, 9,10) On June 20, 2011, the State of New Jersey reached a settlement with 3 companies wherein they would pay a total of 15 million dollars for chromium contamination site clean-up. This amount cannot begin to address the cost of remediating the environmental damage. (11)

In 2003 and 2004, Brick Township in Ocean County was ranked as the second safest city in the United States. However, this township has been in the news since for a claimed autism epidemic in which 40 children out of over 6,000 were found to be autistic. Many of the autistic children were born in northern New Jersey, the hub of the chromate industry. (11) French's landfill in Brick Township has been closed and designated as an EPA hazardous Superfund Site. Chromium, arsenic, cadmium, mercury, and nickel have been found in acreage surrounding the site. The report takes pains to note that the chromium present was *not* of the species VI, or hexavalent, type.(12) The reasons for this are now becoming clear.

The terrible environmental contamination that occurred in French's Landfill was described in a recently-published book on autism and the environment by journalist Brita Belli. (13) Twenty-four worrisome contaminants were listed. Chromium was not one of them. Nor was it mentioned by Belli in the section of her book dealing with autism in New Jersey. I believe that it is the presence of a toxic form of chromium that is largely contributing to the high incidence of autism in New Jersey, and chromium VI is largely the reason why the NJ autism incidence is higher than that of other badly polluted areas of this country in which contaminants similar to the list of twenty-four noted above are also likely present.

The autism epidemic could be the fastest evolving disorder in all of medical science. I stand by my proposition that the record high autism rates in New Jersey are being driven in large part by unrecognized and largely unaddressed exposure to high levels of chromium (VI) in the northern part of the state which also has the highest autism rates. The consequence of this oversight has been additional years of ecosystem damage and human suffering by this extremely toxic and mobile poison. The resolution of this crisis in NJ appears to reside, not in science, but in removing the road blocks obstructing the identification and removal of potent environmental toxins as chromium (VI). Elimination of these barriers set up by powerful commercial and political interests is the crucial first step of remediation, and what must be done if the rate of autism in New Jersey is to be effectively addressed and reversed.

1. **Committee clears 7-bill assembly package to bolster state's response to autism. New Jersey General Assembly. March 5, 2006.**

2. **Augenstein S. The Star-Ledger. March 29, 2012. N.J. Still ranks high in autism, report says. Accessed June 25, 2012.**

3. **City Mayors. The most polluted cities. Http://www.citymayors.com/environment/polluted-uscities.httm. Accessed June 25, 2012**

4. **Autism, Biology and the Environment. In: Science- Based Effective Treatments. 2006 Spring Conference, General Session. Autism Research Institute. San Diego, CA. pp 3-11.**

5. **Burke T, Fagliano J, Goldoft M, et al. Chromite ore processing residue in Hudson County, New Jersey. *Environ Health Perspectives* (92):131- 37, 1991.**

6. **Health Consultation. E.C. Electroplating (a/k/aGarfield Chromium Groundwater Contamination Site). Garfield, Bergen County, New Jersey. N.J. Department of Health and Senior Services. April 26, 2010.**

7. **Nagourney SJ, Wilson SA, Buckley BB, et al. Development of a standard reference material for Cr(VI) in contaminated soil. *J Anal AT Spectrom.* 2008/DOI: 10.1039/b808488b / Technical Note. Accessed June 25, 2012.**

8. **Lane A. Weakened Rules a Boon to 3 Polluters. Newark Star Ledger. Mar 7, 2004.**

9. Michaels D. *Doubt is Their Product: How Industries' Assault on Science Threatens Your Health.* Cambridge MA. Oxford University Press. Cambridge. 2008.

10. Mc Garrity TO, Wagner WE. *Bending Science: How Special Interests Corrupt Public Health Research.* Cambridge, MA. Harvard University Press. 2008.

11. http://www.morris.patch.com/.../honeywell-to-pay-millions-for-chromium-clean... Accessed June 25, 2012.

12. Brick Township, New Jersey. http://en.wikipedia.ord/wiki/Brick Township, New Jersey. Accessed June 25, 2012.

13. Belli Brita. *The Autism Puzzle.* New York: Seven Stories Press; 2012:49-60.

13. Landfill Information. In:http://www.twp.brick.nj.us/content.ask?ContentId+569. Accessed June 25, 2012.

Appendix C

HOW WE HARM OUR LIVERS

Air, water pollution,
-dark skies, dirty water

Gut-derived toxins
-the enemy within

Food additives

Heavy metals

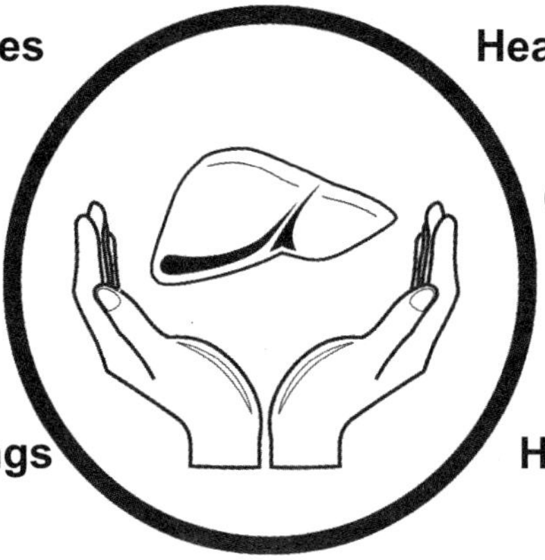

Alcohol

Cigarettes

Pesticides

Stress

Toxic buildings

Herbicides

Prescriptions, over the counter medications

Biotoxins from electromagnetic fields*

High fat and sugar foods

"Love your liver and live longer," Dr. Cabot says.

*Dr. Dietrich Klinghardt's Fundamental Teachings-Mercola.com

Appendix D

Suggestions for newborn testing, based on biochemical and immune abnormalities affecting liver function

Readers Please note:

These investigations appear here for review by experts. Some of these tests are not currently commercially available. Autism is such a complex and poorly understood entity that even if all of these tests were completed and the results found to be normal, there is still no guarantee an adverse vaccination reaction would not occur.

1. Methylenetetrahydrofolate reductase (MTHFR) testing for C677T and A1298C mutations.
2. Urine malondialdehyde (MDA) to assess free-radical damage to body lipids (including those in the brain).
3. Measure blood reduced glutathione by speciated isotope dilution mass spectrometry.*
4. Urine pyroglutamate in organic acid test to assess intactness of glutathione recycling.
5. Urinary dihydroascorbic acid to ascorbic acid ratio to check body's antioxidant capacity.
6. Measure blood for oxalates (Ref 39 of book), or natural killer cell function. (www.scia.com)

*This method corrects for interspecies conversions of glutathione due to oxidation and provides accurate, precise measurement of both oxidized and reduced forms, allowing construction of a useful ratio between the two.

7. Measurement of urine gluteo-, gliado- & caseomorphins.

8. Documentation of low secretory immunoglobulin A (IgA) levels in mother's breast milk. Absence of breast feeding would, by definition, count as a positive test.**

9. Genomic testing ,including liver cytochrome p450 subtypes, genetic methylation variants, and apolipoprotein-E after establishment of normal ranges for infants.***

**CDC researchers report rotavirus vaccine did not "take" well in breastfed infants from India. They attributed this vaccination failure to the demonstrated presence of high levels of IgA in breast milk.(1)

From this finding, one may hypothesize that a low level of IgA in breast milk --as is found in U.S. mothers-- or deprivation of breast feeding altogether, may result in damage to the infant's immature immune system by overloading it with standard doses of multiple vaccinations administered simultaneously. This condition could be aggravated by the presence of maternal selective IgA deficiency, a relatively common inherited condition.(2)

(1)Moon SS, Wang Y, Shane AL et al. Inhibitory effect of breast milk on infectivity of love oral rotavitus vaccines. *Pediatr Infect Dis J*, 2010 Oct 29 (10):919-923.

(2)http://www.immunedisease.com/about-pi/.../selective-iga-deficiency.html.

*** Cost of genomic testing would have to decrease substantially to make this a viable test option.

Appendix E

Nutritional Analyses of Various Sea Vegetables

	Calories	Fat	Carbohydrate	Protein	Fiber	Calcium	Potassium	Magnesium	Phosphorous	Iron	Sodium
	cal/100g	g/100g	g/100g	g/100g	g/100g	mg/100g	mg/100g	mg/100g	mg/100g	mg/100g	mg/100g
ALARIA (Alaria esculenta)	262	3.6	39.8	17.7	38.5	1,100	7,460	918	503	18.1	4,240
DULSE (Palmaria palmata)	264	1.7	44.6	21.5	33.3	213	7,820	271	408	33.1	1,740
KELP (Laminaria longicruris)	241	2.4	39.3	16.1	32.5	942	11,200	900	423	42.6	4,460
LAVER (Porphyra umbilicalis)	318	4.5	45.1	28.4	30.3	188	2,680	378	408	20.9	1,610
HIZIKI (Hizikia fusiforme)	236	0.8	47.3	10.0	17.0	1,400	14,860		59	29.0	
ARAME (Eisenia bicyclis)	267	1.3	51.8	12.0	7.0	1,170	3,860			12.0	
KOMBU (Laminaria japonica)	259	1.1	54.9	7.3	3.0	800	5,800		150	15.0	
WAKAME (Undaria pinnatifida)	271	1.5	51.4	13.0	4.0	1,300	1,800		260	13.0	1,100
NORI (Porphyra tenera)	322	0.7	45.0	34.0	7.0	470	330**		380	23.0	
ROCKWEED (Ascophyllum nodosum)	241	1.0	52.0	10.0	6.0	4,200	2,300	600	200	50.0	3,700
BLADDERWRACK (Fucus vesiculosis)	276	3.6	54.9	6.0	3.8	2,200	2,260	660	90	36.0	2,710
Recommended Daily Allowances (RDAs)	2,000+	65+	300+	50+	25+	1000 mg	3500 mg	400 mg	1,000 mg	18 mg	2,400 mg

+ These guidelines are set by the USDA and the US Dept of Health and Human Services.

Most nutritional assays for North Atlantic sea vegetables provided by Maine Coast Sea Vegetables

Most nutritional assays for Japanese sea vegetables taken from *Vegetables From the Sea*, S.&T. Arasaki, Japan Publications, 1983.

All assays, particularly iodine, vary widely by season, drying method, storage method, etc.

RDAs are determined by the National Academy of Sciences and subject to periodic revision. See www.nas.edu

g/ 100g=grams per 100 grams
mg/ 100g=milligrams per 100 grams
mcg (micrograms)=milligrams per kilogram
100 grams = 3.5 ounces
I.U.=International Units

Nutritional Analyses of Various Sea Vegetables

	Iodine	Manganese	Copper	Chromium	Fluoride	Zinc	Vit. A*	Vit. B_1*	Vit. B_2*	Vit. B_3*	Vit. B_6*	Vit. B_{12}*	Vit. C	Vit. E
	mg/100g	mg/100g	mg/100g	mg/100g	mg/100g	mg/100g	IU/100g	mg/100g	mg/100g	mg/100g	mg/100g	mcg/100g	mg/100g	IU/100g
ALARIA	16.6	1.02	0.172	0.21	4.3	3.44	8,487	0.558	2.73	10.5	6.23	5.03	5.9	4.92
DULSE	5.2	1.14	0.376	0.15	5.3	2.86	663	0.073	1.91	1.89	8.99	6.6	6.34	1.71
KELP	45.3	1.23	0.148	0.24	3.9	2.86	561	0.549	2.48	3.62	8.63	2.6	4.16	2.71
LAVER	1.4	3.46	0.612	0.12	5.8	4.15	4,286	0.577	2.93	5.92	11.21	17.5	12.03	5.09
HIZIKI	40						150	0.01	0.20	4.6		0.57		
ARAME	98-564						50	0.02	0.02	2.6				
KOMBU	193-471	1.67					430	0.08	0.32	1.8	0.27	0.3	11.0	
WAKAME	18-35	3.05					140	0.11	0.14	10.0		.6*	15.0	
NORI	0.5	2.04					10,000	0.21	1.00	3.0	1.04	13-29	20.0	
ROCKWEED	153.7	23.3	0.21	0.058		1			0.50	18.2			37.5	
BLADDERWRACK	65	6.7	0.3	0.2		1.3								
Recommended Daily Allowances (RDAs)	150 mcg	2 mg	2 mg	12 mcg	1.5 mg	15 mg	5,000	1.5 mg	1.7 mg	20 mg	2 mg	6 mcg	60 mg	30 I.U.
								*(Thiamine)	*(Riboflavin)	*(Niacin)	*(Pyrodoxine)	*(Cyanocobalamin)		

Most nutritional assays for North Atlantic sea vegetables provided by Maine Coast Sea Vegetables

Most nutritional assays for Japanese sea vegetables taken from Vegetables From the Sea, S.&T. Arasaki, Japan Publications, 1983.

All assays, particularly iodine, vary widely by season, drying method, storage method, etc.

RDAs are determined by the National Academy of Sciences and subject to periodic revision. See www.nas.edu

g/ 100g=grams per 100 grams
mg/ 100g=milligrams per 100 grams
mcg (micrograms)=milligrams per kilogram
100 grams = 3.5 ounces
I.U.=International Units

From Sea Vegetables Celebration. **Book Publishing Co. Used with permission**

If mankind can change its ways

and autism is ended

we will forever sing His praise

for lives that have mended.

MDA 21 November, 2011

BOOK ORDERING INFORMATION

(1) Printed copies available from:
WWW.AMAZON.COM

(2) e-Publication: i-Bookstore -accessible with i-Pads, i-Phones, and i-Pods ® (planned for 2013)

(3) Printed copies from the website:

www.autismatabbasplace.com

book cost: $19.95

***Shipping and handling (U.S.A.): $5.00**

Michigan residents add: $1.50 sales tax

Method of payment: PayPal or money order

(no personal checks please)

***International orders see website for rates.**

***Shipping rates subject to change without notice.**

G.U.D. Publishers

P.O. Box 268

Cedar, MI 49621-268

231-228-4567